MARKETING
FOR PHARMACISTS
2nd Edition

Notice

The author and the publisher have made every effort to ensure the accuracy and completeness of the information presented in this book. However, the author and the publisher cannot be held responsible for the continued currency of the information, any inadvertent errors or omissions, or the application of this information. Therefore, the author and the publisher shall have no liability to any person or entity with regard to claims, loss, or damage caused or alleged to be caused, directly or indirectly, by the use of information contained herein.

MARKETING
FOR PHARMACISTS
2nd Edition

DAVID A. HOLDFORD, RPH, MS, PHD

Associate Professor
Virginia Commonwealth University School of Pharmacy
Medical College of Virginia Campus
Richmond, Virginia

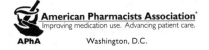

American Pharmacists Association®
Improving medication use. Advancing patient care.
APhA   Washington, D.C.

Editor: Nancy Tarleton Landis
Acquiring Editor: Sandra J. Cannon
Indexer: Suzanne R. Peake
Layout and Graphics: Roy Barnhill
Cover Design: Scott Neitzke

© 2007 by the American Pharmacists Association
APhA was founded in 1852 as the American Pharmaceutical Association.

Published by the American Pharmacists Association
1100 15th Street, NW, Suite 400
Washington, DC 20005-1707

To comment on this book via e-mail, send your message to the publisher
at aphabooks@aphanet.org.

Library of Congress Cataloging-in-Publication Data

Holdford, David A.
  Marketing for pharmacists / David A. Holdford. -- 2nd ed.
    p. ; cm.
  Includes bibliographical references and index.
  ISBN 978-1-58212-106-2
1. Pharmacy--Practice. 2. Marketing. I. Title.
  [DNLM: 1. Community Pharmacy Services. 2. Marketing--methods.
QV 737 H727m 2007]

  RS100.H65 2007
  615'.10688--dc22

                                        2007022388

This book is dedicated with love to my parents,
Arthur and Dorothy.

Contents

Preface

Marketing for Pharmacists was written for student pharmacists, practicing pharmacists, and pharmacy managers who want a basic introduction to the concepts of marketing pharmacy products and pharmacists' services. Like the first edition, this second edition emphasizes the marketing of pharmacists' services, although it does include some discussion of the marketing of drugs and pharmacy merchandise. The primary purpose of the book is to expose students, pharmacists, and pharmacy managers to techniques and ideas that can make them more effective in meeting the needs and wants of their patients.

Marketing for Pharmacists consists of 13 chapters divided into six sections: Foundations of Marketing, Marketing Pharmacist Services, Consumer Behavior, Marketing Strategy, Segmentation and Promotion, and Pricing and Placing Pharmacist Services. The book is designed to be easily accessible to people without a business background. Nevertheless, it can also benefit those who have substantial experience and training in business.

WHY A MARKETING BOOK FOR PHARMACISTS?

Pharmacy leaders and educators have been telling pharmacists and students for years that they need to alter current methods of practice and help forge new professional models within the dynamic health care environment. However, pharmacists and students who want to bring about change in their practice settings rarely have the experience or training to do so. Often, they find that effecting change in the pharmacy profession can be quite difficult, and they end up settling into old habits of practice.

The practice of marketing is a way to bring about change. *Marketing for Pharmacists* presents the concept of marketing at the level of the individual employee in a hospital or community setting. In contrast, most marketing texts address the topic at the corporate level. The premise of this book is that marketing should be performed by every individual in a business or organization, not just by a corporate department. Pharmacists can use marketing to build their practices, develop and provide innovative services, and generate business for their employers or organizations.

WHO CAN USE THIS BOOK AND HOW?

The book is designed to be used by student pharmacists, educators, practicing pharmacists, and pharmacy managers. Pharmacists and managers can read the book from beginning to end, or they can jump to topics of interest. I recommend that pharmacists who are not familiar with marketing concepts read the first two chapters, on basic marketing terms and concepts.

Pharmacy educators can use the book, in required or elective courses, to teach students the basics of marketing. *Marketing for Pharmacists* can be used as a text for a broad range of required courses, such as introduction to community pharmacy practice, implementing pharmaceutical care, and managing pharmacist services. Alternatively, the book can be used for elective or graduate courses in pharmaceutical marketing.

The chapters cite many references to articles that illustrate the concepts discussed, and I encourage readers to look for some of those articles. Educators, in particular, can use the referenced articles to supplement information in the chapters and to promote class discussion.

OBJECTIVES

Pharmacists, students, and managers who read this book should gain an appreciation for the need to market pharmacist services and a basic understanding of the principles and terminology of marketing. They should be able to list and discuss important elements of excellent pharmacist services, suggest different methods for designing and providing pharmacist services, delineate processes through which consumers choose and evaluate pharmacy products and pharmacist services, develop a marketing plan, recognize different marketing strategies and understand their advantages and disadvantages, suggest ways to segment markets for pharmacist services, develop a promotional plan, propose innovative pricing tactics not commonly seen in pharmacy practice, and understand pharmaceutical channels of distribution.

Ultimately, the purpose of this book is to teach students and pharmacists to

- Lead change within their work setting,
- Avoid complacency,
- Take chances,
- Look outside the door of their pharmacy,
- Assess their practice setting,
- Be optimistic,
- Use their imagination to better serve patients, and
- Effectively articulate their value to all customers.

Acknowledgments

This book owes a great deal to pioneering pharmacy scholars who taught and conducted research in the field of pharmaceutical marketing. These scholars include Mickey Smith, Dev Pathak, Joe Wiederholt, Marv Shepherd, Norm Carroll, Jean Gagnon, Albert Wertheimer, Arthur Nelson, Dale Christensen, Dennis Tootelian, Dave Kreling, and Ray Gosselin. The book also recognizes and incorporates the work of their successors in the pharmacy marketing field: Karen Farris, Bill Doucette, Earlene Lipowski, Bruce Berger, Richard Hansen, Doug Ried, Mike Rupp, Bonnie Svarstad, Jeanine Mount, Anandi Law, Jan Kavookjian, Jon Schommer, John Bentley, Woodie Zachry, Suzan Kucukarslan, Charles Phillips, Stephanie Crawford, Donna West, David Tipton, Ken Lawson, Richard Cline, Julie Ganther-Urmie, Marcia Worley, Tim Stratton, Randy McDonough, Sheryl Szeinbach, and many more.

I am especially indebted to Norm Carroll, who read and commented on chapters 1 through 11 and wrote chapters 12 and 13. I have been very fortunate to have Norm, an expert in pricing and channels of distribution, as a colleague at Virginia Commonwealth University.

PART I

FOUNDATIONS
OF MARKETING

INTRODUCTION TO MARKETING

Objectives

After studying this chapter, the reader should be able to

- ❏ Define the term *marketing*.
- ❏ Describe four key elements associated with the act of marketing.
- ❏ Compare and contrast transactional marketing and relationship marketing.
- ❏ Analyze some of the misconceptions surrounding the practice of marketing.
- ❏ Justify the need for pharmacists to market themselves and their services.
- ❏ Describe major trends having an impact on the practice of pharmacy.
- ❏ Differentiate various approaches to marketing from the "marketing concept."
- ❏ Assess key obstacles to the marketing of pharmacists' professional services.

A patient tells the pharmacist at a community pharmacy that he wants to quit smoking but does not think he has the willpower to do so. After asking several questions to assess the patient's readiness, the pharmacist concludes that he could quit successfully, given the right therapeutic strategy. She encourages the patient to enroll in the pharmacy's smoking cessation program.

A second-year pharmacy student has decided to become a faculty professor specializing in community pharmacy. The student knows that faculty positions can be very competitive and wants to maximize his chance of success. He develops a plan that will enable him to gain the right set of skills and experiences to market himself for a faculty position.

A hospital wants to open an outpatient satellite pharmacy to serve patients in another part of the metropolitan area. The assistant pharmacy director is asked what services the satellite pharmacy might successfully provide. The assistant director's first step is to identify physicians who practice near the proposed satellite and pay them a visit.

A pharmacist believes her patients would benefit if the pharmacy offered women's health services. However, her immediate supervisor is resistant to change and unlikely to support anything that will make his life more complicated. The pharmacist begins to investigate what resources would be necessary to start a women's health clinic and what strategies she might use to reduce her manager's objections.

In each of these four scenarios, the pharmacist or future pharmacist can solve a problem through the application of marketing methods. This chapter will help readers begin to understand such marketing problems.

The purpose of the chapter is to define the term *marketing*, describe key elements of any marketing problem, and explain the importance of effective marketing to pharmacists and student pharmacists. The chapter will clarify misconceptions about marketing and illustrate different marketing approaches. Finally, it will identify and discuss key problems that pharmacists face in marketing their services.

WHAT IS MARKETING?

Marketing is a discipline that promotes the resolution of problems by identifying and meeting the needs of customers. In pharmacy practice, the customers served by marketing may be patients, physicians, nurses, or anyone else who interacts with pharmacists. Marketing can be formally defined as exchanges between people in which something of value is traded for the purpose of satisfying needs and wants. Key elements of this definition are *people, value, needs and wants,* and *exchange.*[1]

People. Marketing is an act between people. The discipline is concerned with human behavior and draws upon the behavioral sciences (e.g., psychology, sociology, and anthropology) to solve marketing problems. Marketers who understand the causes of human behavior can effectively influence others.

> *The customers served by marketing may be patients, physicians, nurses, or anyone else who interacts with pharmacists.*

Value. Marketing deals with transactions of value. Valued items are not necessarily money or tangible products; people often trade money and other forms of wealth for intangible things such as information. The valued item exchanged can be anything that might meet a need or want, including money, material, labor, information, and ideas.

Needs and wants. Marketing is concerned with satisfying the needs and wants of customers. Needs are things necessary for survival, such as food, water, clothing, transportation, and shelter. Wants are things that are desired but not absolutely essential for survival. People frequently confuse needs and wants. A person may say that he "needs" a Mercedes-Benz automobile, but what he is really saying is that he wants one, since his need for transportation can be met in many other ways. The person who says he needs a Mercedes-Benz is expressing a preference or want for one specific mode of transportation over another.

Exchange. For the process of marketing to occur, there must be an exchange or the potential for an exchange. Without an exchange of something of value, needs or wants cannot be satisfied.

MARKETING EXCHANGES

Marketing exchanges can be viewed as discrete or continuous. At its most extreme, a discrete exchange is an isolated, individual transaction involving people who never expect to do business again. In contrast, continuous exchanges are a series of transactions taking place over time. How a marketer views exchanges helps determine how he or she practices marketing.

Marketers who view exchanges as discrete, unrelated events tend to practice *transactional marketing*. Here, it is important to drive a hard bargain in every transaction because the marketer assumes there is a single opportunity to maximize profit. The goal is to "win" the transaction by getting as much as possible while giving as little as possible in return. Since the parties involved do not expect to ever do business again, there is no concern about future exchanges, customer satisfaction, or customer loyalty to the business.

Marketers who view exchanges as a continuous series of transactions over time practice *relationship marketing*. The parties in such exchanges focus less on "winning" the transaction and more on serving the needs of the other party. The aim is transactions that satisfy both parties and result in future business. These marketers believe that cultivating relationships with customers will have greater long-term benefits than would a purely transactional approach to marketing.

As a marketing strategy, relationship marketing can be used to serve targeted groups of patients,[2] but it can also be adopted as a philosophy of practice. Most pharmacists would agree that the relationship marketing approach better serves the health care needs of patients. Often, however, pharmacists practice as transactional marketers, focusing on completing the sale and getting the patient out the door.

Pharmacists who practice relationship marketing see each service interaction as one step in the process of building a professional or therapeutic relationship with an individual. They view each occasion to speak with a patient, physician, payer, nurse, or member of the general public as an opportunity to establish or strengthen a relationship.

For example, telephoning a physician to make a therapeutic recommendation can be viewed as a single event or as one in a series of events over time. A pharmacist with a transactional viewpoint is concerned only with completing the call and getting on with work. The outcome of the call is less important than the desire to conclude it as quickly as possible.

When the pharmacist has a relationship viewpoint, the objectives for the telephone call change. The first and most obvious objective is to get the physician to accept the recommendation. A second, less obvious objective is to establish or maintain the pharmacist's credibility as a source of future therapy recommendations. Even if the physician does not accept the pharmacist's immediate recommendation, the pharmacist can lay the groundwork for acceptance of future recommendations. Pharmacists who practice relationship marketing take each exchange seriously, realizing that one bad interaction with a patient or health care professional can hurt future ones.

EVERY PHARMACIST IS A MARKETER

When we take the broad view that marketing consists of exchanges of things of value between people, it becomes clear that any activity directed toward meeting people's needs and wants is a marketing activity. Thus, pharmacists who engage in any of the following actions are involved in marketing:

- Dispensing a prescription drug,
- Assisting patients in the selection of nonprescription medications,
- Providing drug information to patients or health care professionals,
- Taking a patient's blood pressure,
- Counseling patients about drug regimens,
- Convincing key decision makers of the benefits of pharmaceutical care,
- Looking for employment,
- Recruiting pharmacists for a new job, and
- Educating student pharmacists.

With this broad definition of marketing, nearly everything pharmacists do in their jobs is a marketing activity. Therefore, to be successful in pharmacy, pharmacists need to be good marketers.

Marketing is about influencing others. It is finding out what people need and want and getting them to take actions to meet those needs and wants (e.g., make a purchase, take their medicine as directed). Marketing pharmaceutical services is about influencing the following people:

- *Patients.* Pharmacists persuade patients to take their medicines as directed, use nonprescription medicines appropriately, follow instructions, monitor their therapy, and pay for a higher level of services.
- *Physicians.* Pharmacists influence physician behavior through persuasive conversations and written communications.
- *Third-party insurance companies.* Pharmacists try to persuade third-party insurance companies to pay higher dispensing fees and reimburse pharmacists for cognitive services.
- *The public.* Pharmacists promote an image of professionalism and trust to the general public.
- *The pharmacist's employer.* Pharmacists induce employers to hire them rather than one of the many other pharmacists competing for a job. Once in a position, pharmacists must constantly demonstrate their value to their employer.
- *The pharmacist's boss.* Pharmacists encourage their bosses to manage differently, to try new ways of meeting the needs of patients, and to maximize rewards for good work.
- *The pharmacist's co-workers.* Pharmacists influence co-workers when they sell them on new ideas, get them to participate in group projects, and motivate them to handle a fair share of the workload.

WHY MARKETING IS IMPORTANT TO PHARMACISTS

Given the current strong demand for pharmacists and the increasing prescription workload, the prospects for pharmacy may seem bright. But the profession may be in a struggle for its future. The U.S. health care system has limited resources for managing the nation's health. Health care providers (e.g., physicians, nurses, hospitals, managed care organizations) are all competing for a portion of those resources. Providers who demonstrate and promote their value are more likely to thrive in the future health care environment.

No one knows what the future will bring to the pharmacy profession. All we know is that things are going to change. To understand what changes may occur, it is useful to look at the recent past.

In 1980, life for the average pharmacist was quite different from what it is today. Pharmacists had more time to spend with patients. They were not under such intense pressure to fill large numbers of prescrip-

> *Marketing is a proven tool for influencing change.*

tions. Most patients paid for prescriptions out of their own pockets, and their daily lives did not seem so rushed. Mail order pharmacies were rare, and Internet pharmacies were almost 20 years in the future. The concepts of managed care and pharmacy benefit managers (PBMs) were relatively new. The terms disease state management, medication therapy management, and pharmaceutical care had not been invented.

Times have changed. Now, pharmacists are in an extremely competitive health care market. They compete with each other and with other health care professionals for opportunities to meet patients' needs. They are continually pressured to increase their productivity by using technology and technician help, while at the same time filling increasing numbers of prescriptions. Many pharmacists say they feel stressed and dissatisfied in their current practice settings.

These changes have not always benefited patients. In many cases, pharmacists have cut back the time they spend helping patients with drug-related problems. Substantial numbers of preventable medication errors have occurred. Noncompliance with medication regimens is a serious problem. Although patients generally express satisfaction with pharmacists and pharmacy services, their health care needs often are not being met.

Pharmacists have a choice: They can allow things to continue on the present course, or they can try to implement change. If new pharmacist graduates choose not to become involved in influencing the course of their profession, they can expect to spend approximately 40 years in a career in which their work lives are determined by the whims of others. Pharmacists can choose to be passive about their future work lives, or they can take control over their lives, their careers, and their profession. Marketing is a proven tool for influencing change.

There are tremendous opportunities for pharmacists who are willing to adapt to and influence change in health care. To grab these opportunities, pharmacists need to control their practice instead of letting others do so. One way is to take a more active role in marketing pharmaceutical services and promoting their value to patients, physicians, insurers, and other important decision makers. It may be nice to reminisce about the good old days of the community pharmacist, but reminiscing will not bring back the past. Pharmacists need to deal instead with the present and future practice of pharmacy.

IMPACT OF SOCIETAL TRENDS

Although it is impossible to foretell the future, it is certain that major societal trends will influence the practice of pharmacy. Some trends that will pose challenges to the profession are discussed in the following paragraphs.

Consumer-directed health care (CDHC). CDHC is a health insurance strategy that encourages greater patient involvement in health care purchasing decisions. Patients are asked to take greater financial responsibility for their health care choices through the use of co-payments, co-insurance, high-deductible health insurance plans (HDHPs), and health savings accounts (HSAs). HSAs are tax-sheltered accounts similar to individual retirement accounts and are typically used in combination with HDHPs to pay for qualified medical expenses for individuals and their families. Money contributed over the years to HSAs and left unspent at retirement can be used for nonhealth expenses without penalty. Just as important, CDHC empowers patients to manage their health through disease management, wellness programs, preventive care, self-monitoring technology, and medical education Web sites. The idea behind CDHC is that consumers will make better health choices if they have the right incentives and information. As CDHC spreads, pharmacists will find opportunities to demonstrate their value by assisting consumers with their health decisions.

Aging baby boomers. For the post-World War II baby boom generation now facing retirement, that transition will be different than it was for their parents. Boomers are accustomed to leading active lives and demanding much of themselves and society. They are unlikely to accept the status quo in health care. Rather, they can be expected to demand drugs and services not just to treat illness but to enhance lifestyle. Boomers will want pharmacists to help them live longer and healthier lives. If pharmacists do not meet this demand, boomers will find others who will.

Around-the-clock society. Today, people operate in a 24/7/365 environment, and they expect services and products to be available at any time of the day or night. Offering convenience is no longer an option for pharmacies; it is essential for competing in the market. The key will be to develop pharmacy systems that not only offer convenience but also ensure appropriate drug use and prescribing.

Improvements in service technology. Many of the manual and repetitive tasks involved in pharmacy practice can now be performed with robotic and self-service technology. This poses a threat to pharmacists who are unwilling to change their practice by providing higher levels of professional services. Conversely, innovative pharmacists see this as a tremendous opportunity to better serve their patients.

Budgetary constraints. Demands for public and private funding of health care are competing with other societal priorities. Since the 1990s, health care spending in the United States has increased at a higher rate than population growth, general inflation, and gross domestic product. This has placed an increased financial burden on households, businesses, and local, state, and federal government and forced them to make hard choices about how to spend their budgeted dollars. If the rise in health care spending continues unchecked, it will require major shifts in funding away from other important societal needs. Money that is spent on the health care needs of an aging population, advances in health care technology, compliance with new treatment guidelines, and health care inflation cannot be spent on transportation infrastructure, energy, housing, interest on debt, Social Security, maintenance of the military, protection of the environment, and other competing responsibilities. The budgetary constraints on health care purchasers will force pharmacists to compete with providers such as nurses, physicians, allied health professionals, and health educators for the available health care dollars.

Health care innovations. Innovations in health care will affect pharmacy practice. Advances in human DNA mapping and genetic profiling have led to a new area of research and therapy, pharmacogenomics. This new field promises to explain the influence of genetic differences on patient response to drugs and lead to the development of treatments specific to an individual's genetic makeup. In oncology, for instance, genetic testing has been used to target breast cancer patients who are most likely to benefit from trastuzumab, a monoclonal antibody. Other advances will come from the field of nanomedicine, in which tiny "machines" at the molecular level can be used to diagnose and treat medical conditions. Nanotechnology holds potential for the development of molecules that deliver chemotherapy agents or other drugs to targeted sites, minimizing common adverse effects. Tiny machines may also repair damaged tissue in skin, bone, and internal organs.

Rising global competition. Health care competition is becoming global as providers in countries such as Thailand, India, Malaysia, Mexico, and Canada compete with U.S. providers. Patients who lack health insurance or have high-deductible coverage are seeking high quality, low-cost care across our borders. This trend, called medical tourism, is small but growing. As the patient's share of medical costs increases, more individuals may seek providers globally for surgical procedures, drugs, and other health care. With growing pressure to contain costs, some health care jobs may be outsourced to non-U.S. providers, following the current example of radiological services.

RESPONDING TO PHARMACIST SKEPTICISM ABOUT MARKETING

Pharmacists are often reluctant to become involved in marketing, in large part because of the generally low public opinion of marketers. When asked what marketing is, the average pharmacist is likely to mention intrusive telephone solicitation, pushy salespeople, or irritating television and radio advertisements. When asked about the purpose of marketing, the average pharmacist probably would talk about selling and promoting soap and automobiles, not health care.

Pharmacists and student pharmacists may also be skeptical about the relevance of marketing for pharmacists. Their skepticism may arise from misconceptions about marketing. Many people think of marketers as unethical people who intrude on your life, disturb your dinner with phone calls, clutter the landscape with advertising, and interrupt your favorite TV and radio shows to entice you to buy things you don't want. In truth, marketing is often practiced that way.

Many criticisms of marketers are well deserved. Some marketers operate with the attitude that pursuit of profit is paramount and any action that maximizes shareholder equity is acceptable. Deceit, misinformation, and dishonesty are often tolerated when they increase sales revenue. Unethical marketers may even find it acceptable to put consumers at risk (e.g., by selling faulty or dangerous products). Their rule of conduct is caveat emptor—let the buyer beware. It is little wonder that the public has a general distrust and low opinion of marketing.

In truth, unethical and abusive business practices have tarnished the public's image of marketing. High-pressure selling can force customers to make purchases under stress. Deceptive advertising misleads consumers about product features and attributes. Bait-and-switch sales promote low-price offerings, with the intent of selling the customer a higher-priced item. Consumer privacy is frequently violated through unwanted e-mail, telemarketing, and junk mail and the sale of personal information. Planned obsolescence results in products of lower quality that will need to be replaced more frequently, resulting in more sales.

But not all marketing is like that. The following examples show how marketing can be used for good.

- Pharmacists and other health care professionals at Sentara Healthcare in the Norfolk, Virginia, region developed and implemented a marketing plan to teach consumers why antibiotics should not be used to treat colds and other viral infections.

- Pharmacists use marketing methods in "academic detailing" to influence physician prescribing patterns and to counteract the influence of drug company marketing programs.
- Throughout the United States, pharmacists provide disease management services, therapeutic monitoring, vaccine administration, collaborative practices with physicians, and a variety of other advanced clinical services. The most successful services are provided by pharmacists who are good marketers.
- Worldwide, pharmacists are participating in international programs in family planning, smoking cessation, alleviation of hunger and childhood diseases, and prevention and treatment of HIV/AIDS—most of which use social marketing strategies to succeed.

MISCONCEPTIONS ABOUT MARKETING

A pharmacist may think, "Why do I need marketing? I'm a pharmacist (or will be one soon). I don't want to be some fast-talking used-car salesman. I want to save lives and improve patients' quality of life, not peddle my services to customers. Pharmacy is a health care profession. It has a higher purpose and is above the need for (ugh!) marketing. Besides, I plan to work in clinical pharmacy, where marketing isn't important. If not, I'll work for an employer who will handle all that marketing stuff for me. Marketing has very little applicability to my current or future practice."

The following misconceptions about marketing are common among pharmacists and student pharmacists:

1. *Marketing is selling.* As shown in Figure 1-1, selling is just one function associated with marketing. Other marketing functions include researching customer needs and wants, developing strategies, maintaining customer records, delivering products and services, financing, promotion, pricing, and monitoring customer satisfaction. Selling is completing a sale. Marketing covers the sale as well as all the activities before and after the sale. Marketing activities can begin before a need is identified and continue long after that need is satisfied.
2. *Marketing is bad.* Some critics charge that marketing is inherently bad because it results in socially undesirable actions such as overconsumption, waste, and the purchase of products that people would do better without (e.g., cigarettes). Although it is accurate to say that marketing can promote socially negative acts, it is also true that marketing can be used to promote positive behaviors. For example, marketing has been used to promote AIDS prevention, smoking cessation, birth control, and other preventive health behaviors. Although we may dislike the

FIGURE 1-1 Some marketing functions.

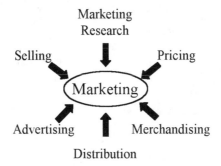

marketing of some products (e.g., liquor and cigarettes), ethical marketing practices benefit society.
3. *Health care professionals do not need to market.* If you look at successful health care professionals, be they physicians, nurse practitioners, optometrists, dentists, or pharmacists in any setting, you will see that they excel at marketing. They may just call it something else.
4. *Employee pharmacists in community pharmacies do not need to market.* Most employee pharmacists have a great deal of autonomy in how they practice, with relatively little oversight from their bosses. In many cases, these pharmacists are responsible and held accountable for the success of their practice sites. Upper management may provide support services such as TV or newspaper advertising or research about the local market, but in the end, most marketing in pharmacy is conducted by individual pharmacists through the services they provide and the personal relationships they develop with their patients.
5. *Only community pharmacists need to market.* All pharmacists need to market themselves and their ideas. Hospital, managed care, long-term care, and government pharmacists need to market their programs to physicians, nurses, administrators, payers, and the public. Meeting the needs of these "customers" entails many of the same marketing methods that are used with patients.

A basic premise of this book is that all pharmacists can use marketing as a tool to help others. Like any tool, marketing can help when used appropriately and hurt when misused.

APPROACHES TO MARKETING

The manner in which pharmacists approach marketing problems determines how marketing benefits patients. Pharmacists choose their marketing strategies on the basis of their assumptions about the relative

TABLE 1-1   Approaches to Marketing

Approach	Driving Force	Philosophy
Production approach	Production	Be fast and cheap.
Sales approach	Promotion	Be fast and cheap and promote it extensively.
Product approach	The product idea	If you build it, they will come.
"I'm the expert" approach	Expert opinion	I know what is best for you.
Marketing concept	Needs and wants of customers	How can I help you?
Societal marketing concept	Needs and wants of customers and society	How can we make the world a better place to live?

importance of (1) the pharmacy business, (2) the customers or patients, and (3) society. In other words, marketing can emphasize the pharmacy business and profitability, patient well-being, or the overall impact on society. A pharmacist's marketing approach balances the often conflicting concerns of these three constituencies. The following sections describe different approaches pharmacists can take to marketing problems (Table 1-1).[1]

Production Approach

The production approach to marketing holds that the major task of an organization is to pursue efficiency in production and distribution. The primary goal is an organization that runs smoothly. The assumption is that cheap and efficient provision of goods and services is sufficient for success in business. Little explicit consideration is given to the needs and wants of patients and society. The production approach assumes that if products and services are cheap enough, customers and society will demand them.

A pharmacy that takes a production approach to the provision of services may attempt to fill as many prescriptions as possible, without consideration of whether consumers benefit from the prescriptions. Such a pharmacy treats patients not as individuals but as units of production; the more units that travel through the process, the better. This may seem to be a foolish way of doing business, but some pharmacies do use this approach.

A drawback with the production approach is that firms compete almost entirely on the basis of price and availability. The goal is to produce as much as possible as cheaply as possible. The assumption is that people will buy anything if it is cheap enough. But the fact that something is produced and available does not mean that customers will want it and be willing to pay for it.

Another problem with the production approach is that someone can always provide cheaper products and services. Decades ago, community pharmacists who competed solely on price were underpriced by chain pharmacies that were able to take advantage of economies of scale. Some chain pharmacies were later underpriced by mail order pharmacies that were able to centralize the filling of prescriptions and did not need to maintain stores in the community. The lesson to be learned is that low price and availability are often not sufficient for survival in the market.

Sales Approach

The sales approach is only a little more sophisticated than the production approach, although it recognizes that production and distribution are not enough for success. Selling effort—the use of advertising, sales discounts, personal selling, and promotions that increase demand for a product or service—is also crucial. Selling effort combined with cheap production and distribution is most closely associated with mass marketing, which attempts to sell to very large markets.

As with the production approach, the primary goal of the sales approach is to sell as much as possible, with little explicit consideration of the customer's needs and wants. With the sales approach, any sale is a good sale.

Aggressive application of the sales approach is one reason for the public's negative opinion of and adversarial relationship with marketers. Tactics such as those used by aggressive telephone salespeople have caused consumers to go to great lengths to avoid their calls, such as using answering machines to screen calls, taking legal action, and lobbying for legislative relief.

The sales approach also can promote unnecessary sales, such as selling people products they do not want. In pharmacy practice, this approach can be damaging to the patient, since it can encourage patients to use unneeded and even harmful drugs.

Product Approach

In the product approach, marketers become so passionate about a product or service that they are blind to the need for and market viability of the product or service. Products and services may be of very high quality—which may be more than customers need or want. Typically, products are conceptualized and designed without much input from the customer. The philosophy of the product approach is, "If you build it, they will come." This can cause a narrow-mindedness that leads marketers to place the needs of the product over the realities of the market.

Not to be confused with the production approach, the product approach assumes that a business that develops a better product will automatically find consumers who will buy it. It has been said that if a man builds a better mousetrap, the world will beat a path to his door. But often this doesn't happen. Even the best new products entering the market can fail. They can be too expensive, poorly promoted, difficult to find and purchase, or of higher quality than customers need or want.

Furthermore, incremental improvements in established products frequently overshoot the needs of consumers. Many products fail because their quality exceeds the needs of most people in the market. This provides opportunities for disruptive innovations—simpler and less expensive alternatives—to fill the gap.[3] In health care, retail clinics (e.g., the "minute-clinic") have sprung up to compete with physician offices by providing cheaper and more convenient, but less comprehensive, service to patients suffering from minor ailments.

Pharmaceutical care is a product with which the pharmacy profession has become enamored. But the fact that it is a good idea does not mean it will be a success. Clearly, it can benefit many patients, but pharmaceutical care is a higher quality of service than patients are accustomed to. Input must be solicited from patients to customize pharmaceutical care to individual patient needs and desires. A pharmacist who expects patients to accept and pay for pharmaceutical care but does not use effective marketing is practicing the product approach.

"I'm the Expert" Approach

This approach holds that the provider knows what is best for the customer and it is the customer's responsibility to comply with the provider's decisions. The "I'm the expert" approach frequently overlaps with the product approach to marketing. Both are paternalistic; they do not include the customer in decision-making. Health care professionals often use this approach when providing care. They think their many years of education make them more qualified to decide a patient's treatment.

The Marketing Concept

The best approach to marketing asserts that the main task of an organization is to determine the needs and wants of targeted customers and satisfy them through the design, communication, pricing, and delivery of appropriate and competitive products and services. This approach, called *the marketing concept,* has several distinguishing features. First, in designing, promoting, and delivering products and services, it explicitly considers the viewpoints of customers. This means that the customer drives decisions about marketing strategy—not the product, provider, production, or sales. Second, the marketing concept focuses on targeted customers; marketers match their products and services to those customers whom marketers can serve better than their competitors can. Targeting recognizes that circumstances do not necessarily support every idea and venture, so marketers need to focus on meeting the needs of select customers. Finally, customer satisfaction is a goal of the marketing concept. Customers are satisfied when they perceive that their needs are being met.

Societal Marketing Concept

The societal marketing concept is an extension of the marketing concept that includes consideration of the needs and wants of society along with those of individual consumers. The societal concept originated because of the potentially negative consequences of strictly observing the marketing concept; a single-minded focus on satisfying individuals can hurt others.

For pharmacists, a strict interpretation of the marketing concept means that they satisfy patients and payers of drug products. But doing so can have a negative societal impact. An extreme example is that of a drug addict. Satisfying a drug addict may mean giving drugs on demand. This may not be in the best interest of either society or the drug addict. Similarly, a patient may be satisfied with fast, cheap, and friendly service, but that may not always be in the patient's or society's best interest.

Discussion of the marketing concept in this book will consider the impact of marketing on society. When pharmacists adopt the marketing concept in their provision of services, they seek to satisfy the needs and wants not only of their immediate patients but also of society.

PROBLEMS ASSOCIATED WITH MARKETING PHARMACIST SERVICES

It would be wonderful if the public recognized and fully appreciated the contributions of pharmacists—and equally wonderful if pharmacists could practice in the manner promoted by the profession. However, pharmacists function in the real world, where the practice of pharmacy is constrained by a number of realities. Some of the realities that must be overcome before pharmacists can reach their full professional potential are described in the following sections.

Control of Practice by Nonpharmacists

Unlike many other professionals in the United States, pharmacists have limited control of how their profession is practiced. Pharmacist control over the profession has gradually decreased as corporate ownership of pharmacies has increased. In the past, pharmacy ownership was limited to licensed pharmacists; today, most pharmacies are controlled by corporate entities. These corporations are answerable to shareholders and often are run by nonpharmacists.

With corporate ownership, the primary job of pharmacy managers is to enhance shareholder value. Therefore, corporate managers make decisions based on profit, a framework that is not always consistent with the goal of enhancing patients' health and well-being. When a pharmacist must choose between filling prescriptions (which generates revenue) and counseling or therapeutic problem solving (neither of which typically generates revenue), it is easy to see the conflict.

Nonpharmacist owners are also less likely to appreciate the problems associated with inappropriate drug use. They lack the training, experience, and professional socialization to fully grasp many of the issues facing pharmacy practitioners. Nonpharmacist owners are likely to be distracted by nonpharmacy concerns within the business. Prescription drugs are only a small portion of the overall business in many large corporations, especially mass merchandisers and grocery stores. Corporate owners may consider the practice-related concerns of pharmacists to be of minor consequence.

Product Orientation

Most pharmacists in the United States work in community pharmacies that use a retail business model. The retail business model revolves around selling merchandise. Service is a major component of retailing, but the success or failure of retail businesses ultimately depends on the sale of tangible goods.

The product focus of the community pharmacy model contrasts with the professional service model found in medicine, law, and other professions. The professional service model is typically oriented toward information and counseling. Revenue is generated from these activities. This contrasts with the retail business model, in which revenue comes from providing a broad range of merchandise for customers in a convenient manner.

Conflicting Professional and Merchant Roles

The pharmacy profession and pharmacists must often struggle to balance their professional and merchant roles. Pharmacists are responsible for making a profit as well as for helping patients with their health-related needs. This balancing act can cause conflict.

Pharmacists must generate revenue by filling more prescriptions. Time that is not spent filling prescriptions (e.g., time spent on patient counseling and disease management activities) does not usually generate revenue. However, pharmacists have a professional responsibility to monitor patient therapy, educate and counsel patients, and solve therapeutic problems even if no revenue is generated. These are the professional activities that can truly improve patient health and quality of life. Most pharmacists face this struggle daily.

Poorly Defined Public Image of Pharmacists

Although the public's image of pharmacists is generally favorable, most consumers do not have a clearly defined image of what a pharmacist does. Ask a person on the street what a pharmacist does, and the person is likely to say something vague about dispensing medicines. It is unlikely that the person will know anything about the details of the tasks involved in dispensing.

In addition to their general lack of awareness of pharmacists' responsibilities, consumers have limited expectations of pharmacists. Research has demonstrated that patients are unaware of the services pharmacists are able to provide and unlikely to appreciate the roles and responsibilities of pharmacists.[4]

Silos of Health Care

The U.S. health care system is largely made up separate "silos" of providers and payers who work independently without much consideration of how they fit within a system of care. Decisions about medications often focus on containing costs instead of improving the overall quality and value that drug products bring to the health care system. Incentives for pharmacists typically ignore pharmacists' potential to improve patient outcomes and instead highlight low costs, convenience, and speed of service.

Pharmacist Shortages

As this book is being written, many areas of the United States do not have enough trained pharmacists to meet the demand. This has caused a strain on the provision of pharmaceutical services. In these locations, pharmacists struggle just to provide basic dispensing services. Given the current workload, clinical services are not even a consideration for some pharmacists.

The shortage of pharmacists can be problematic for the marketing of pharmaceutical services. If pharmacists do not have sufficient time and resources to explore new opportunities, those opportunities will be put on hold, and competing providers such as nurse practitioners or physician assistants may step in to fill the void.

> *Pharmaceutical marketing is not just about selling drugs. It is also about promoting new ideas.*

However, there can be a positive side to the pharmacist shortage. It can give pharmacists the ability to influence their practice settings and spend more time on professional duties. Competition for pharmacists makes it possible for the most competent, talented pharmacists to negotiate better working conditions, including the ability to provide clinical services. Employers are more likely to take a chance on clinical services if it means keeping top pharmacists. In addition, the pharmacist shortage makes it more economical to support pharmacists with technology and technician help. This can permit pharmacists to delegate tedious nonprofessional tasks.

SUMMARY

Pharmaceutical marketing is not just about selling drugs. It is also about promoting new ideas. Marketing can further the idea that pharmacists provide value and should receive compensation for professional services. It can help pharmacists exert influence over the way pharmacy is practiced.

Marketing can be used to solve almost any problem in pharmacy. It can be used in personal career management, in influencing change in practice settings, and in enhancing job effectiveness. Marketing can help persuade patients to adhere to medication plans, physicians to prescribe medicines appropriately, and management to support pharmacy practice initiatives. It can be used to recruit good employees, attract and keep patients, provide innovative services, and compete with other professions for a portion of the health care pie.

This book focuses on marketing ideas and methods that can be used by pharmacists. It is based on the premise that marketing is not just a corporate activity but an activity that needs to be practiced by every pharmacist.

By reading this book and applying its lessons in practice, pharmacists can develop a "marketing mindset."[5] Such a mindset helps the pharmacist to systematically consider a series of important issues (e.g., Who are my customers?) before implementing any initiative to serve patients. It creates a shift in thinking from "What is wrong with patients, physicians, nurses, and payers? Why don't they appreciate my contributions? Why won't they listen to my recommendations?" to "How can I improve my services? How can I develop a message to communicate their value? What can I do to make my services more useful and desirable to customers than those of my competitors?"

References

1. Kotler P. *Marketing Management: Analysis, Planning, and Control.* 4th ed. Englewood Cliffs, NJ: Prentice Hall; 1980.
2. Doucette WR, McDonough RP. Beyond the 4P's: using relationship marketing to build value and demand for pharmacy services. *J Am Pharm Assoc.* 2002;42:183–93.
3. Christensen CM, Bohmer R, Kenagy J. Will disruptive innovations cure health care? *Harv Bus Rev.* 2000;78(5):102–12.
4. Chewning B, Schommer JC. Increasing clients' knowledge of community pharmacists' roles. *Pharm Res.* 1996;13(9):1299–304.
5. Quinn G, Albrecht T, Marshall R, et al. "Thinking like a marketer": training for a shift in the mindset of the public health workforce. *Health Promot Pract.* 2005;6(2):157–63.

Additional Readings

Kennedy DT, Small RE. Development and implementation of a smoking cessation clinic in community pharmacy practice. *J Am Pharm Assoc.* 2002;42:83–92.

Painter N. Establishing a clinical practice. Advice for new practitioners. *Am J Health Syst Pharm.* 2006;33:519–20.

Smith NC. Marketing strategies for the ethics era. *Sloan Manag Rev.* 1995 (summer):85-97.

Solomon DK. Marketing hospital pharmacy services. *J Res Pharm Econ.* 1989; 1(2):119–29.

Stevenson J. Persuasion as a strategy for managing up. *Am J Health Syst Pharm.* 2001;58:S4–S6.

Exercises and Questions

1. List specific examples of how marketers have intruded into your life, irritated you, or deceived you. Compare those with examples of how marketers have made your life better. What differentiates the "bad" marketers from the "good" ones?
2. Think about a pharmacist who you believe has an excellent reputation among patients and co-workers. What behaviors does this person engage in to develop such a positive image? Would you consider this person to be a good marketer? Why or why not?

3. Will Rogers, famous cowboy philosopher, has been quoted as saying, "Let advertisers spend the same amount of money improving their product that they do on advertising, and they wouldn't have to advertise it." Do you agree or disagree with this? Why?
4. How might pharmacists use marketing to
   a. Enhance their personal career opportunities?
   b. Provide better care for patients?
   c. Promote a positive image of pharmacists among the public?
5. What major barriers do pharmacists face in providing clinical services such as diabetes management in your practice setting?
6. List things of value that are exchanged between pharmacists and patients, physicians, and nurses.
7. Review the section in this chapter titled "Problems Associated with Marketing Pharmacist Services." Which of these problems do you think is the greatest barrier to the progress of the profession? Why? How can pharmacists overcome this barrier?

Activity

Identify an issue in the professional pharmacy literature or on a professional association Web site that might be marketing related. Describe the issue and why you think it relates to marketing.

2

IMPORTANT MARKETING CONCEPTS

Objectives

After studying this chapter, the reader should be able to

❑ Define the following marketing terms: *product; core, expected, and augmented product; marketing myopia; potential, target, and actual markets; the marketing mix; the four P's; positioning.*
❑ Describe two major categories of competitors.
❑ Differentiate internal from external customers.
❑ Explain the difference between the "products" of pharmaceutical care and of dispensing activities mandated by OBRA '90 legislation.
❑ Identify and differentiate the various marketing tasks, the type of demand they regulate, and suggested strategies.

Alfreds is a new discount department store chain that recently entered the market in the Mid-Atlantic States. This regional chain has 125 stores in 12 states. Forty of the stores have pharmacies, and more pharmacies are planned for the next 2 years.

Alfreds advertising literature describes a customer-friendly attitude: "We consider our customers to be our guests." Alfreds tries to provide high-quality products at low prices. The stores offer a wide range of merchandise, including snack bar items; school and office supplies; stationery and party favors; hardware; apparel for men, women, and children; small appliances; jewelry and accessories; home decorating supplies; housewares and commodities; health and beauty aids; candy and snack foods; cameras and electronics; pet supplies; prescription and nonprescription drugs; bathroom accessories, bedding, window treatments, and rugs; and furniture and lighting. The stores are well-lighted and convenient, and service is fast and friendly.

One metropolitan area has five Alfreds stores, the first of which opened in April 2000. Each of these stores has a pharmacy that provides basic dispensing services. Alfreds management wants to use these five stores to develop pharmaceutical care models of practice that can be implemented throughout the chain. Alfreds and a local school of pharmacy have reached a collaborative agreement to promote the practice of pharmaceutical care in the area. Alfreds will fund a full-time clinical faculty member from the school to oversee the implementation of pharmaceutical care in each individual store and to create quality clerkship rotation sites for PharmD students.

The faculty member, Dr. Lina Kennedy, wants her first project at Alfreds to have a major impact on patient care. Her success in the effort hinges on an understanding of the marketing problem at hand, the resources available, and the environment in which the program will be implemented. She needs to answer the following questions:

1. What is the product I will be offering? What will make it stand out from what pharmacists are now doing in the community?
2. Who are my customers and competitors? What patient groups (e.g., market segments) might benefit most from a pharmaceutical care program?
3. How strong is the market for my product? What is the market for pharmaceutical care? What might I do to expand the market?

The purpose of this chapter is to define marketing terms and ideas that every pharmacist and pharmacy manager should know. Pharmacists who understand the correct use of marketing terminology will be better able to communicate their ideas in language that can be understood by managers, marketers, and others.

The "Alfreds" vignette describes Dr. Kennedy's marketing problem. It touches on some basic marketing concepts—product, customers, competitors, and market—that pharmacists need to understand and address in order to market their services.

DEFINING THE PRODUCT

In the factory we make cosmetics; in the drugstore we sell hope.

—Charles Revson, founder of Revlon Cosmetics

A product is defined by nonmarketers as some tangible object that is sold for and bought with money. Examples include automobiles, furniture, clothing, books, and drugs.

Marketers define the term more broadly. A concise and widely recognized definition of a product is "anything of value that can be exchanged to satisfy a need or want."[1] According to this definition, a product can be an object (e.g., a syringe of antibiotic), a service (e.g., cholesterol screening), an activity (e.g., a poison prevention campaign), a person (e.g., Bob, the clinical pharmacist), a place (e.g., a Medicine Shoppe pharmacy), an organization (e.g., the American Pharmacists Association), or a concept (e.g., pharmaceutical care). Each is valued and satisfies needs or wants. For example, Bob, the clinical pharmacist, offers solutions to the needs of his employer and the patients he serves. The American Pharmacists Association offers benefits to its members and the profession as a whole.

How pharmacists define their product is critically important, because it specifies the ultimate purpose of pharmacists and frames the way in which they approach pharmacy problems. In other words, the way pharmacists define their product shapes their priorities and actions. If pharmacists define their product as the provision of a drug, then they fit the "count and pour, lick and stick" and "pill pusher" labels that some people associate with pharmacists. These pharmacists practice a production approach to marketing, in which they focus on the provision of a tangible product (i.e., a physical object).

However, people pay for the benefits of drugs, not the tangible drug product. Patients, insurers, and other purchasers pay for the positive health outcomes that drugs can bring, such as pain relief, quick recuperation from illness, reduced risk of death, and improved quality of life. The tangible drug is just a vehicle for delivering health benefits associated with the drug.

Drugs by themselves rarely bring about health benefits. Indeed, a patient can be harmed if she does not know how to take the drug appropriately. Pharmacists who fixate on the provision of a tangible drug suffer from what marketers call *marketing myopia*. Marketing myopia is shortsightedness on the part of marketers who become preoccupied with selling the tangible product while failing to consider the needs of the consumer.[2] Marketing myopia exists when pharmacists see themselves as providers of drugs rather than managers of drug-related health outcomes.

To prevent marketing myopia, the *total product concept* was introduced.[3] This concept (Figure 2-1) looks at a product in terms of three primary components: (1) the core product, (2) the expected product, and (3) the augmented product.

The *core product* (center circle in Figure 2-1) is the benefit resulting from the bundle of tangible goods, information, and services. It meets

FIGURE 2-1   The total product concept. (Compiled from reference 3.)

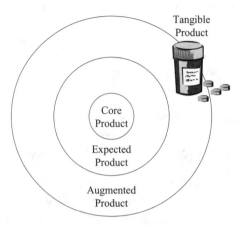

the underlying need that the overall product package satisfies. It is what the customer is really buying. The woman who purchases a camera is not buying a mechanical box; she is buying pleasure, nostalgia, and a form of immortality.[1] The middle-aged man who buys a sports car is not buying a means of transportation; he is buying memories of youth and the hope to relive them. For customers of pharmaceutical services, the core product may be health related (e.g., improved quality of life) or not (e.g., greater peace of mind, a feeling of control over one's illness).

The next circle in the total product concept is the *expected product*. The expected product is what the customer expects to receive from a marketer. The expected product is situation specific; it varies according to the circumstances and the people involved. In most pharmacy dispensing situations, the patient expects only to receive the correct drug in an accurately labeled container within a reasonable time period. In other circumstances, high levels of pharmaceutical services have trained patients to expect more.

Anything provided that is beyond what the customer expected is called the *augmented product*. The augmented product is the bundle of tangible product(s), information, and services that exceeds the customer's minimal expectations. The augmented product is also called the *differentiated product* because it differentiates one business from the next. Things that might augment community pharmacy services include counseling, therapeutic monitoring, insurance assistance, free home delivery, blood pressure monitoring, refill reminders, telephone and Internet refills, selection of nonprescription medications, patient package inserts, compliance programs, drive-through services, and disease management services.

The expected product and augmented product provide a bundle of benefits that result in the core product. A pharmacy's bundle of services and merchandise is meant to fulfill patients' health care and non-health care needs. The more a patient perceives the benefit bundle as unique and valuable, the more likely it is that the patient will patronize the pharmacy.

> *How a pharmacy differentiates its product from those of competitors determines the relative value to the patient.*

In reality, no bundle of services and merchandise offered by any pharmacy is exactly like any other (e.g., no two pharmacies are likely to be equally convenient), although the patient may perceive pharmacies as interchangeable. How a pharmacy differentiates its product from those of competitors determines the relative value to the patient. If a pharmacy wants to attract and keep patients, its differentiated product should offer greater value in their eyes.

DIFFERENTIATING PHARMACEUTICAL CARE FROM BASIC DISPENSING

Many pharmacists and student pharmacists have difficulty explaining the difference between pharmaceutical care and typical dispensing activities in a way that others can understand. It is easy to identify activities associated with pharmaceutical care, such as therapeutic monitoring and disease management services, but it is difficult to interpret these in a way that friends or family can fully comprehend. This is a serious problem, because payers and patients often believe that services commonly associated with pharmaceutical care are covered by dispensing fees. In truth, dispensing fees cover only the minimum level of service that pharmacists are capable of providing. If pharmacists want to expand their service compensation beyond dispensing fees, they must be able to articulate the differences. This section describes how pharmaceutical care can be differentiated from basic dispensing services.[4]

Services associated with pharmaceutical care differ from normal dispensing activities because they exceed the services mandated and paid for under the Omnibus Budget Reconciliation Act of 1990 (OBRA '90). That legislation contains requirements for dispensing outpatient prescription drugs covered by Medicaid. OBRA '90 standards have been adopted as minimum requirements for most pharmacist services in prescription benefit plans and have thus been established as a minimum standard of practice in community pharmacy. OBRA '90 requires that pharmacists accurately dispense a drug requested on a prescription order, clarify incomplete or illegible prescriptions, *not* dispense any order that a reasonable and prudent pharmacist would recognize as containing an obvious error, keep patient profiles, carry out drug-use review (DUR) activities, and offer to counsel Medicaid patients about using their medications.[5] Medicaid dispensing fees, where applicable, pay for these services.

OBRA '90 requirements represent only the minimum level of services that pharmacists must provide to patients. They are far below what pharmacists are capable of providing. OBRA '90 requires only that pharmacists "offer to counsel." A half-hearted offer can meet the requirements of the law but does little to encourage a productive discussion about the patient's drug therapy.

To meet OBRA '90 therapy review requirements, pharmacists need only assess the medication records for the most flagrant errors. However, many drug-related problems are not readily evident without some research. This research, conducted by those who practice pharmaceutical care, often requires better patient records, more in-depth interviewing and counseling, and more extensive problem solving than what is mandated by OBRA '90.

Pharmaceutical care focuses on drug-related problems, not drugs. These drug-related problems may or may not be associated with the dispensing of a prescription. Cognitive services associated with pharmaceutical care include activities such as[6]

- Patient consultation to discuss the patient's expectations and concerns about his or her drug therapy, evaluate the patient's understanding of the drug therapy, collect information from the patient, and identify the patient's drug-related needs.
- Pharmacist assessment of the patient's drug therapy to identify current or potential problems.
- Development of care plans to establish specific goals, monitoring schedules, and a written patient record.
- Patient education, recommendations, and referrals that will provide individualized, current information about the patient's drug therapy; give instructions for proper use of medications; demonstrate special techniques or devices (e.g., the proper use of inhalation devices); and provide health and disease information.
- Patient monitoring and follow-up at planned intervals to ensure that new drug therapy problems do not develop, therapeutic goals are being met, and actual patient outcomes are evaluated and documented.

OBRA '90 does not require in-depth examination of drug-related problems. Patient counseling under OBRA '90 consists of reviewing only basic facts about a prescription, such as how to take and store the medication.

Activities not covered by OBRA '90 include consultations with patients, prescribers, or other health care providers; detecting therapies that are "safe" but less than optimal either therapeutically or economically; selecting the appropriate drug product (e.g., interchange among generically, pharmaceutically, or therapeutically equivalent products); training patients to use blood-glucose-monitoring devices; and conducting "brown bag" drug review sessions where patients bring in all of their medications from home for examination.[5]

The distinction between cognitive services and OBRA '90-mandated services is highlighted when the pharmacist detects therapy that does not cost-effectively achieve the desired outcome but is not so clearly in error that the pharmacist must refuse to dispense the drug.[5] The time, effort, and skills required to pursue this type of drug-related problem are not covered by the normal dispensing fee. However, pursuing such problems can improve the quality of care and reduce overall health care costs.

Medication therapy management (MTM) is an alternative description of pharmaceutical care. The concept originated in discussions among professional organizations before passage of the Medicare Prescription Drug Improvement and Modernization Act of 2003. Eleven organizations representing all areas of pharmacy practice agreed on a formal definition of MTM. Although MTM is similar to pharmaceutical care, the concept has the advantage of formal recognition by the federal government and acceptance by all major pharmacy organizations as an essential element of drug therapy. Government recognition of MTM was a key step toward federal compensation of pharmacists for professional services. Although MTM is quickly becoming the preferred term for intensive clinical pharmacist services, this text will continue to use the term pharmaceutical care.

DETERMINING THE MARKET

To the average person, *market* refers to a physical place where buyers and sellers gather to exchange goods and services. To a marketer, the term means the set of all individuals and organizations who are actual and potential buyers of a product or service. A market consists of anyone who might conceivably buy a given product.[1]

A market includes actual and potential buyers. Actual buyers are current customers. Potential buyers are people or groups who might have (1) a real or unrealized interest in products or services and (2) the means to acquire them.

By this definition, wherever there is potential for trade, there is a market. This point is illustrated by the story of an American shoe company that sent a new, inexperienced salesman to one of the South Sea Islands to see if there was a market for shoes.[1] The salesman came back disappointed and declared, "The people on the island don't wear shoes. There is no market there." The chief executive was skeptical about the new salesman's conclusion, so he sent his

> *Since anyone who consumes pharmaceuticals may also benefit from monitoring, counseling, and drug information, the potential market for pharmaceutical care is quite large.*

ace salesman to the island. The day after arriving, the ace salesman called back exclaiming, "The people on the island don't wear shoes. There is a tremendous market here."

The first salesman limited his market definition to current users of the product. The second salesman's definition included everyone who had two feet and might eventually be interested in shoes. This story has a lesson for pharmacists: Pharmacists who perceive their market as only current customers overlook opportunities to expand their market.

Figure 2-2 demonstrates the relationship between the total population and the *potential market* for pharmaceutical care. For many products, the potential market is only a fraction of the overall population within a given area. This is not the case in pharmacy, because the potential market for pharmaceutical services includes anyone who might conceivably use drugs. Since anyone who consumes pharmaceuticals may also benefit from monitoring, counseling, and drug information, the potential market for pharmaceutical care is quite large.

Within the potential market are the *target market* and the *actual market*. The target market consists of those people in the potential market who are most attractive to the marketers. These people might be targeted because they are most profitable or best suited to the capabilities of the marketer. The target market is the focus of marketing efforts.

The actual market is those people who actually consume products or services. It is typically much smaller than the target market and may even include individuals outside the target market. Its size depends on how well a marketer succeeds in attracting and keeping customers within a market. The actual market for products depends on the customer's

1. *Level of interest.* Customers must be aware of a product and recognize a need for it.
2. *Necessary resources.* Customers must be able to pay for the product.
3. *Willingness to pay.* Customers must be willing to pay for the product.

FIGURE 2-2 Comparison of potential, target, and actual markets for pharmaceutical care.

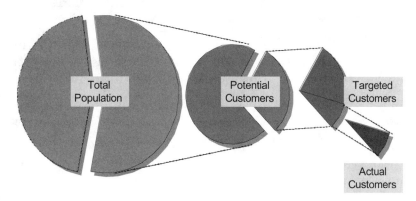

For higher levels of pharmacist services such as pharmaceutical care, the target and actual markets are likely to be smaller than the potential market. The target market is smaller because some patients may not currently need intensive pharmacist services and because providing such services may not be profitable, given the lack of compensation by prescription drug insurers. The actual market for these services may be further limited if people are (1) unfamiliar with the availability of pharmaceutical care, (2) unaware of their need for it, (3) unwilling to pay for it, or (4) unable to pay for it.

Therefore, for pharmaceutical care to achieve its market potential, pharmacists must

- Identify people in the population who might benefit from pharmaceutical care (i.e., the potential market),
- Identify and attract people in the potential market who best match the services that pharmacists can provide (i.e., the target market), and
- Serve those customers who have sufficient interest and resources to pay for it (i.e., the actual market).

THE MARKETING MIX

The term *marketing mix* describes the actions that can be taken by marketers to attract and keep customers. The marketing mix is popularly known as the *four P's* of product, price, promotion, and place. Businesses compete with each other by offering some combination of product, price, promotion, and place designed to cause customers to choose their product over a competitor's.

TABLE 2-1   Elements of the Marketing Mix for a Prescription Drug

Product	Price	Promotion	Place
Fast, friendly service	Dispensing fee	Advertising	Easy access
Extensive selection of	Percentage of	Direct	to the
herbal and	average	marketing	pharmacist
nonprescription products	wholesale	Public relations	by telephone,
and general merchandise	price	Personal	Internet, or
Disease management	Insurance	selling	in person
services	coverage	Sales	Convenient
Generic drugs	Co-payment	promotion	location and
Computerized patient	Professional	Word-of-	parking
profiles	service fee	mouth	Delivery and
Pleasant service	Financing	promotion	mail services
surroundings			offered
Competent, empathetic,			
and reliable care			

The product is the array of tangible goods, services, and information offered, as described earlier in this chapter. The price is what is asked of customers in exchange for the product. Promotion refers to communications designed to inform, persuade, and remind customers about the product. Place is the manner, location, and ease of access to the product.

The marketing mix for a prescription drug consists of elements of the four P's that differentiate one pharmacy from another. Table 2-1 lists elements of the marketing mix associated with the dispensing of a prescription drug.

To address unique elements of the marketing mix associated with services, some service marketers have expanded the four P's to seven P's. The three extra P's associated with services are physical evidence, participants, and process. *Physical evidence* refers to the physical environment in which services are provided and all tangible cues (e.g., employee dress, documentation, signage). Physical evidence is related to place; it includes elements associated with the location of the service, such as the parking lot and physical building. *Participants* are all personnel associated with the provision of services, including both providers and customers. Participants are related to product and promotion. *Process* includes all policies, procedures, rules, guidelines, and workflow design associated with the provision of services. Process is most closely related to product.

An additional P, *positioning*, is mentioned by some marketers. Positioning refers to the development of a favorable image in the minds of customers. The position of a product in the mind of the customer is determined by virtually anything the customer sees, hears, smells, tastes, and touches relating to that product. The product itself and how it is priced, promoted, and delivered determine its image in the mind of a customer.

Although the extra P's of physical evidence, participants, process, and positioning may help draw attention to factors of importance to marketers, all of them can be viewed as falling within the traditional four elements of the marketing mix. Therefore, for the sake of simplicity, this book describes the marketing mix in terms of the original four P's: product, price, promotion, and place.

IDENTIFYING COMPETITORS

In most circumstances, pharmacists compete with others to serve customers. It is rare for a pharmacist or pharmacy to have a monopoly on the market, so it is important to identify competitors. Once identified, these competitors need to be challenged in the market. Awareness and understanding of competitors is crucial, because all elements of the marketing mix are assembled with an eye toward these competitors.

Identification of competitors requires a clear definition of one's market or markets. Pharmacists and pharmacies often serve multiple markets. Community pharmacies might serve the prescription drug, cosmetics, photographic, and convenience food markets, as well as many others. A pharmacy's competitors for the prescription drug market may be different from its competitors for the other markets.

Competitors can be divided into two categories.[1] Those in the first category, *intratype competitors,* compete by providing the same or similar products. Examples of intratype competitors in the automobile market are General Motors and Ford. Examples in fast food include McDonald's and Burger King. In community pharmacy, Walgreens, Rite Aid, Eckerds, and CVS are intratype competitors.

Those in the second category, *intertype competitors,* compete by providing distinctly different products that nevertheless meet similar customer needs and wants. Examples of intertype competitors in the evening entertainment market include cinemas, television, restaurants, and local sporting events. Each offers a completely unique product to meet the entertainment needs of consumers. Examples of intertype competitors in other markets include airline and railroad travel, mail and Internet communication, and pharmaceuticals and complementary medicine.

Intratype competitors compete by offering similar tangible and augmented products. They are more immediate threats than intertype competitors, because they compete openly and directly for customers. Intratype competitors are likely to be perceived as substitutes by customers, which makes competition for customers more acute.

TABLE 2-2 Relationship of Competitors to Product Definition

Product Definition	Competitors
Filling a prescription	CVS, Walgreens, Rite Aid, Kroger, Wal-Mart, independents Dispensing physicians Robotic dispensing machines Mail order and Internet pharmacies
One step in a process of purchasing household products, groceries, and prescription drugs	CVS, Walgreens, Rite Aid, Kroger, Wal-Mart, independents 7-Eleven, Quickie Mart Any other general merchandise store without a pharmacy Mail order and Internet pharmacies
Part of a lifelong process of managing patients' health	CVS, Walgreens, Rite Aid, Kroger, Wal-Mart, independents Physicians, nurses, and other health care professionals Health food stores and providers of complementary medicine Mail order and Internet pharmacies

Intertype competitors compete in terms of the benefits provided (i.e., the core product). Although they are less likely to be perceived as substitutes, they are still competing. In fact, intertype competitors can be more dangerous, because it is easier to overlook them. IBM failed to see the competitive threat personal computers (PCs) posed to its mainframe business because it did not see PCs as direct competition.

To understand their competition, pharmacists need to know how their product is perceived by pharmacy customers. As shown in Table 2-2, the way the product is defined determines who the competitors are. Pharmacies whose product is perceived as "filling a prescription" have different competitors from those whose product is defined as "part of a lifelong process of managing patients' health."

CUSTOMERS OF PHARMACIST SERVICES

Who are the customers of pharmacists? They include not just those who come into the pharmacy, but anyone with whom pharmacists must deal. By this definition, everyone who interacts with pharmacists can be considered a customer.

The External Customer

External customers are the people outside your organization with whom you deal, either face-to-face or over the telephone. They include customers in the traditional sense of the word: the people who purchase your products and services. External customers also include your suppliers, the general public, and anyone else you might interact with outside the organization. Interactions with external customers determine the image of your organization. They can also influence the quality of your product, because external customers are often participants in the provision of services. Imagine trying to encourage patient adherence to medication regimens without patient participation.

The Internal Customer

Your other customers are the people who work inside your company and rely on you for the services and information they need to do their jobs. They are not traditional customers, yet they need the same levels of service that you give your external customers.

This point was brought home to me when I was a pharmacist at a hospital that was attempting to improve the quality of services we provided. We were asked to identify the customers of our pharmacy department. Customers were defined as anyone with whom we had dealings either inside or outside the hospital. One of the things we found is that we did not treat some of our internal customers (e.g., housekeeping and engineering personnel) with the respect that should be accorded a customer. We did not greet them when they came into the pharmacy and often treated them as if they were not even there. When pharmacy personnel started to acknowledge their presence with a "Hi" or "Is there anything we can do to help?" the pharmacy employees found that these simple acts led to better communication with those departments and resulted in much better service for the pharmacy and its external customers.

The Customer Chain

The relationships between internal customers and external customers form what can be called a *customer chain*. The chain consists of all of the links between individuals who provide value to the end customer. For example, a patient may be served by a pharmacist who is served by technicians, managers, insurance companies, suppliers, and more. These people are served in turn by others in the customer chain. Each individual in the chain plays some part in fulfilling the customer's needs. Each interaction is an important link in a chain of events that always ends with the customer (or patient).

Studies have consistently shown that well-treated employees treat customers better.[7,8] The problem is that a frightening percentage of managers and pharmacists do not realize that their co-workers are their internal customers. The term *internal marketing* refers to treating one's employees as one would treat external customers. Internal marketing recognizes that the quality of service provided by employees is a direct reflection of how the employees are treated by their managers.

MARKETING TASKS

Although the process of marketing consists of many activities, the ultimate task of marketing is to influence demand. Marketers influence demand for their products and services through their use of marketing tools such as promotional communications, price, and service. Marketers influence demand in a way that helps achieve specific marketing objectives. This does not always mean *increasing* demand. Many times marketers want to decrease demand or keep it steady. Different situations in which pharmacists or other health care marketers can influence demand are described in Table 2-3.[1]

TABLE 2-3   Marketing Tasks to Influence Demand

Market Condition	Health Care Examples	Marketer's Task	Strategies
Negative demand: Potential customers dislike a product and may go to great lengths to avoid it.	Avoidance of colorectal examinations, even by people at high risk for colon cancer Fear of needles Fear of dental work Concern about adverse effect of vaccinations	Change demand from negative to positive	Provide education or peer-to-peer counseling to overcome misconceptions. Understand that the aversion or fear may be based in complex psychological or social beliefs.
No demand: Customers do not feel a need for the product; they may not dislike it, but they are indifferent or uninterested.	Lack of demand for preventive services Minimal perceived need for medication therapy management services	Stimulate interest in the product	Help customers understand what is missing in their lives, and connect the product's benefits to customers' wants or needs.

TABLE 2-3   Marketing Tasks to Influence Demand (*continued*)

Market Condition	Health Care Examples	Marketer's Task	Strategies
Latent demand: There is a strong need but no product to satisfy it.	Unmet needs for cancer cures, affordable health insurance, easy weight-loss strategies, and medications without adverse effects	Identify the demand, assess its extent in the marketplace, and develop new products or services to meet it	Keep abreast of changes in the marketplace and talk to customers. Imagine new ways to meet demand, as has happened with mail-order, Internet, and drive-through pharmacies.
Declining demand: Demand is falling and the decline is likely to continue. (Most products reach this phase and eventually die.)	Decrease in the number of independent pharmacies	Rejuvenate demand	Revitalize the product by improving it, repackaging it, or promoting it to untapped market segments. Some independents have appealed to nostalgia for the old-time pharmacy by reviving features such as soda fountains.
Irregular demand: Undesirable fluctuations in demand are occurring.	Uneven workload in community pharmacies	Even the demand	Redesign pharmacies; invest in technology; schedule appointments; promote senior discount days.
Full demand: Supply is perfectly balanced with demand.	Examples are rare and fleeting	Maintain balance between supply and demand	Consistently work to maintain quality; keep up with changes in the marketplace and customers' desires; defend your market against competitors.

TABLE 2-3   Marketing Tasks to Influence Demand (*continued*)

Market Condition	Health Care Examples	Marketer's Task	Strategies
Overfull demand: Demand exceeds supply; if prolonged, this situation can cause dissatisfied customers to turn to competitors.	Drug product shortages due to interruptions in the supply or surges in demand Demand for nurses, pharmacists, and other health care professionals	Increase supply or reduce demand	Increase production Raise prices or co-payments; lower quality; reduce convenience; restrict availability through formularies and prior-authorization policies.
Unwholesome demand: Demand that is not in the best interests of society.	Demand for cigarettes, and illicit drugs Demand for alcoholic beverages by underage users	Destroy the demand	Portray the product as undesirable. For example, use the message "Smoking kills" or "Smoking isn't cool" to discourage adolescent tobacco use.

Pharmacists often use academic detailing (also called counterdetailing) to influence demand for drugs.[9] The same kinds of strategies used by pharmaceutical sales representatives are used to encourage appropriate prescribing. Typically, academic detailing consists of a visit by a pharmacist or physician to a prescriber to discuss a specific therapeutic topic. The presentation involves educational aids such as brochures and poster boards. Key messages are highlighted and repeated. Follow-up visits are scheduled to reinforce desired prescribing behavior.

SUMMARY

Knowing marketing terminology helps pharmacists learn marketing concepts. There are important lessons in the use of specific terms. For example, a discussion of intratype and intertype competitors teaches that competition originates not just within one business category or profession; rather, it can arise from any business that seeks to fill the same core needs as your business. Knowing marketing terminology can help pharmacists in speaking with business managers. Most people with a rudimentary business background know and use these terms. An understanding of these terms is necessary background for the later chapters in this book, which explain more complex marketing concepts.

References

1. Kotler P. *Marketing Management: Analysis, Planning, and Control.* 4th ed. Englewood Cliffs, NJ: Prentice Hall; 1980.
2. Levitt T. Marketing myopia. *Harvard Bus Rev.* September–October 1965: 26–44.
3. Levitt T. *The Marketing Imagination.* New York: Collier Macmillan; 1983.
4. Holdford DA. Evaluation of the Adequacy of Current Medicaid Reimbursement Rates as They Relate to Cognitive Services Provided by Pharmacists. Budget Bill item 322 #4b. 1998. (Virginia Department of Medical Assistance Services Study requested by Virginia State Legislature.)
5. Christensen D, Fassett W, Andrews G. A practical billing and payment plan for cognitive services. *Am Pharm.* 1993;NS33:34–40.
6. Tomechko M, Strand L, Morley P, et al. Q and A from the pharmaceutical care project in Minnesota. *Am Pharm.* 1995;NS35:30–9.
7. Berry LL, Parasuraman A. Services marketing starts from within. *Mark Manage.* 1992;1:25–37.
8. Gremler DD, Bitner MJ, Evans KR. The internal service encounter. *Logistics Information Manage.* 1995;8:28–34.
9. Soumerai SB, Avorn J. Principles of educational outreach ('academic detailing') to improve clinical decision making. *JAMA.* 1990;263:549–56.
10. Mendota Healthcare. InstyMeds in the news. Available at: www.instymeds.com. Accessed February 26, 2007.

Additional Readings

Bluml BM. Definition of medication therapy management: Development of professionwide consensus. *J Am Pharm Assoc.* 2005;45:566–72.

Christensen DB, Farris KB. Pharmaceutical care in community pharmacies: practice and research in the US. *Ann Pharmacother.* 2006;40:1400–6.

Keely JL. Pharmacist scope of practice. *Ann Intern Med.* 2002;136:79–85.

Medication therapy management services: a critical review. *J Am Pharm Assoc.* 2005;45:580–7.

Exercises and Questions

1. Define the core, expected, and augmented product marketed by
   a. Your pharmacy to patients.
   b. A student or professional association of your choice to potential members.
   c. You to potential employers.

2. Compare medication therapy management and pharmaceutical care.
3. List the internal and external customers of your pharmacy.
4. List the intratype and intertype competitors of your pharmacy.
5. Give one example of a product or service for which you personally have each of the following:
   a. Negative demand
   b. No demand
   c. Latent demand
   d. Declining demand
   e. Irregular demand
   f. Full demand
   g. Overfull demand
   h. Unwholesome demand
6. Read the following paragraphs.[10] Then discuss whether the technology described competes with or complements pharmacist services as currently practiced in your work setting, and why.

> Pharmacies and physicians' offices across the nation are experimenting with ATM-style machines that dispense prescriptions to patients. Promoted as a convenient alternative to waiting in lines at pharmacies, the technology holds promise as a safe alternative to traditional pharmacist services. Rather than waiting in line for 30 minutes with a sick child, patients can insert a prescription and a credit card into the device and receive the medication immediately.
>
> In some retail locations, the device is located next to the pharmacy department to allow patients to pick up called-in prescription refills. Other pharmacies use the device to fill new prescriptions for patients when the pharmacist is busy or after the pharmacy department is closed. Some doctors' offices and emergency rooms use these devices to enable patients to make only one stop for their health care needs. Advocates argue that the machines, when used in combination with bar code technologies, can help shorten the lines in community pharmacies and reduce medication errors.
>
> The machines read the prescription and verify insurance information. Payment is made with the swipe of a credit card. The device then fills a prescription bottle with the prescribed drug, attaches a label, and dispenses the medication along with written drug information. If desired, patients can pick up a telephone located near the dispenser to speak to a pharmacist on a toll-free, 24-hour help line.

Activities

1. Develop a script for a quick, 30- to 60-second "elevator speech" (see Chapter 11) explaining the difference between pharmaceutical care and traditional pharmacist services as required by OBRA '90. Make a persuasive argument for the value of clinical pharmacist services. Ask another person to comment on your content and delivery.
2. Read the article by Keely listed under Additional Readings. How well did she summarize the scope of practice of pharmacists? Do you think it is acceptable for others to determine our scope of practice? Why?

PART **II**

MARKETING PHARMACIST SERVICES

CHAPTER **3**

CHARACTERISTICS OF SERVICES

Objectives

After studying this chapter, the reader should be able to

❑ Define the following terms: *services, value-added services, pure services.*
❑ Identify four characteristics of services that differentiate them from products.
❑ Discuss how the characteristics of services make them difficult to market.
❑ Describe service categorization methods that can be used to develop strategic insights into the provision of pharmaceutical services.
❑ Apply marketing strategies for dealing with the unique characteristics of services.

"In recent years, the pharmacy profession has attempted to redefine the image of pharmaceutical services in the eyes of patients, payers, and pharmacists. These efforts have promoted the image that pharmacists provide professional pharmaceutical services, not just drugs. A major part of the message is that pharmaceutical services add value to drug therapy. Without the services provided by pharmacists, many drugs can be ineffective and even harmful.

"Efforts to move the image of a profession oriented around drug products toward a service orientation have met with limited success. Although pharmacists are highly trusted, they are still viewed by some in the public and health care community as 'pill pushers' whose primary role is to put pills into a bottle.

"The present image of pharmacists comes from a variety of sources. Promotional messages from professional organizations and pharmacies help shape the view of pharmacists and pharmaceutical services. Forces

45

outside the control of pharmacy institutions, such as the popular media and word-of-mouth recommendations from friends and family, also influence perceptions of pharmacists. Finally, images are shaped by customer experiences with pharmacists. The interaction of pharmacists and customers is especially important in forming perceptions."[1]

Pharmacy is a service profession. Although often associated with a tangible product, pharmacy practice revolves around the provision of services. In fact, there are few instances in pharmacy practice in which services do not accompany a product. Services are provided with every prescription, nonprescription, and nondrug product in the pharmacy. Even basic pharmacy commodities such as generic nonprescription aspirin products require some level of service. At minimum, someone has to stock the shelf.

The importance of service to a business depends on the tangibility of the product offered to customers. The more intangible the offering, the more service oriented a business is.[2] Product-oriented strategies are seen with businesses that provide tangible goods such as salt, soft drinks, and detergents, while service-oriented strategies dominate in businesses that provide intangible services such as investment management, consulting, and teaching. The value provided by service-oriented businesses lies not in tangible things but in information and ideas. Demonstrating the value of intangible offerings requires different strategies than those used for tangible ones.

This chapter discusses the characteristics of services. It differentiates services from products and suggests a number of ways of categorizing services to help pharmacists understand and strategically position their services.

DEFINING SERVICES

Services can be defined as performances or processes that benefit others. Services can accompany a tangible product or be of value by themselves. Those that accompany a tangible product are sometimes called *value-added services.*

Pharmacist services enhance the value of the drug product in a variety of ways. Patient counseling and compliance services increase the effectiveness of drugs. Pharmacist services make pharmaceuticals more accessible, easier to use, and safer. Value-added pharmacy services include most dispensing activities, automated telephone refill programs, assistance with the selection of nonprescription products, and compounding services.

Some services provide value to consumers without a tangible product. These are called *pure services*. Examples are drug information services, poison information services, patient consultations, and disease-screening activities.

Gronroos[3] groups services into three categories on the basis of their utility (i.e., benefit) to the customer: *core services, facilitating services,* and *supporting services.*

> *Services have distinct characteristics that require them to be marketed differently from products such as automobiles and laundry detergent.*

Core services are those that are absolutely essential for the customer to receive a core benefit. A core pharmaceutical service is one that is required for the proper use of medications and optimal patient outcomes. Filling a prescription for a drug to cure a patient's medical condition would be considered a core service. Facilitating services are necessary for the use of core services. Examples in pharmacy are drug inventory control and billing. Without these facilitating services, a needed drug would not be available to dispense. Supporting services differ from core and facilitating services in that they are not essential but can increase the value of the core service and differentiate it from the services of competitors. Supporting services depend on the patient's needs; prescription counseling may fall into this category if the patient is already familiar with the drug and is achieving optimal outcomes with it.

CHARACTERISTICS UNIQUE TO SERVICES

Services have distinct characteristics that require them to be marketed differently from products such as automobiles and laundry detergent.[4] The ways in which services are unique can be described in a framework of four I's:

- *Intangibility.* Services are intangible because they are actions and events. They cannot be seen, held, or touched. Thus, their quality cannot be measured, tested, or verified in advance of the sale to ensure excellence.
- *Inconsistency.* Services are heterogeneous in that no two service performances are exactly alike. They vary from person to person, transaction to transaction, and even time to time. Service quality cannot be easily standardized because of the variations among interactions between buyer and seller.
- *Inventory.* Production and consumption of services are simultaneous. Services are used as they are being produced, or they are not used at all. Once delivered, a service is lost. Services cannot be put on a shelf

for later use. Indeed, if pharmacist counseling services are provided to an inattentive patient, the benefit of that service is lost. The patient must either do without the information or ask the pharmacist to repeat the service.

■ *Inseparability.* The service provider, customers, and service itself are inseparable, because the provider produces the service with the customer's participation. Service quality is determined by both the provider and the customer. In the case of pharmacists' services, patient participation is critical; patients' active role in their therapy is fundamental to pharmaceutical care. Although the patient may not need to be physically present when a prescription is filled, some patient–provider interaction must occur for the patient to receive the product and use it. Even if the prescription is filled in a distant location by an anonymous pharmacist, there is still a patient–provider interaction when the patient reads the prescription and warning labels provided by the pharmacist.

CHALLENGES IN THE MARKETING OF SERVICES

The characteristics of services present special challenges in marketing. Some of these challenges are listed in Table 3-1[5] and discussed in the following sections.

Difficult to Promote

Since services cannot be seen, touched, or sensed, it is difficult to promote their value to others. It is a challenge for marketers to get customers to notice and desire a product they cannot see or touch. To check this for yourself, try to explain to friends and family members the concept of pharmaceutical care and why it is of value. Then have them describe the concept back to you. It is more difficult than it first seems. The intangible nature of pharmaceutical services makes it difficult for consumers to mentally grasp what pharmacists do. It is much easier for consumers to comprehend the purpose of a drug than to comprehend the pharmaceutical services associated with that drug.

Difficult for Customers to Evaluate

The intangibility of services makes them difficult for customers to assess. Some aspects of services are easy to evaluate (e.g., fast, friendly, inexpensive). Other aspects of services are difficult to evaluate even with extensive experience (e.g., clinical skills). For example, it is unlikely that anyone but a pharmacist would be able to recognize when another pharmacist omits critical drug-related information during patient counseling.

TABLE 3-1 Marketing Implications of Characteristics of Services Compared with Goods

Intangibility
Service quality is difficult to assess.
Services cannot be readily displayed or described.
Assigning value and pricing are difficult.

Inconsistency
Employee actions determine the quality of services.
Service quality depends on many uncontrollable factors.
The actual service delivered often does not match what was planned and promoted.

Inventory
Services cannot be stored for later use.
It is difficult to synchronize supply and demand with services.
Services cannot be saved, returned, or resold.
Once services are delivered, they are lost.

Inseparability
Customers participate in and influence the service delivered.
Customers influence each other's service experience.

Source: Reference 5.

In the absence of objective measures of quality, patients use variables that they *can* assess, such as how a pharmacist looks and acts.

Another characteristic of services that makes them difficult to assess is their variability. Service providers such as pharmacists are only human and are subjected to constantly changing circumstances. Each service experience is affected by factors such as the environment (e.g., ringing telephones), the patient (e.g., questions and requests), the pharmacist (e.g., fatigue), and time (e.g., peak commuting time). No one can be certain before visiting a pharmacy what type of service will be experienced.

Often Invisible

Most pharmaceutical services are provided behind the scenes, out of view of the customer. The customer does not see those services and thus cannot appreciate their value unless he or she is made aware of it. Pharmacists who do not inform customers of the "invisible" services they provide get no credit in the eyes of customers for the value they have given.

Supply and Demand Hard to Synchronize

Demand for service is rarely constant in pharmacy settings. Throughout the day and week, there are times when business is relatively slow and other times when it gets quite hectic. It is difficult to synchronize customers' demand for services with the availability of pharmacy personnel to serve them.

The synchronization problem varies by pharmacy setting and type of work provided. In community pharmacies, it is difficult to forecast the demand for services at any specific time. Anyone can walk into a pharmacy at any time and ask for service. Although demand can be regulated somewhat through hours of operation and promotional activities, the demand for service is determined largely by the customer. In hospital inpatient settings, the number of patients is limited, so demand is easier to forecast. Many services such as preparation of intravenous admixtures and distribution of maintenance medications can be performed when demand for more immediate services is low.

CLASSIFICATION OF PHARMACIST SERVICES

Within the pharmacy profession, services are commonly grouped as shown in Table 3-2: by association with a tangible product, by the type of population being served, or by the setting in which services are provided. Although these classifications are useful, they are insufficient to describe the practice of pharmacy in the United States. Classifying services associated with a product says little about how the product is provided and ignores instances in which services may accompany no tangible good (e.g., patient education). Describing services by type of population served does not explain *how* the population is being served. Classifying services according to practice setting makes an implicit assumption that services within each setting are relatively homogeneous; in truth, the levels and types of services provided can vary widely. Pharmacists must look beyond such narrow classifications to recognize innovative ways to serve patients.

Lovelock[6] states that specialization in many service industries has caused inbreeding of ideas and methods. People who work in the hotel, restaurant, and health care industries, for example, tend to remain in these industries for most of their lives. They rely on the same old ways of accomplishing tasks, because they are not exposed to innovative ideas and techniques from other service industries.

Pharmacy is not immune to this inbreeding. Pharmacists and pharmacy managers tend to remain in the profession for most of their lives. They observe the world primarily through the eyes of a pharmacist; consequently, they may overlook opportunities that might be readily apparent to people outside the profession.

Pharmacists might benefit from examining their services and products through new eyes. Pharmacist services can be recategorized according to

TABLE 3-2 Classification of Pharmacist Services

Services Associated with a Tangible Product
Prescription medications
   Refills
   New prescriptions
   Unique administration requirements
    (e.g., intravenous drugs)
Nonprescription medications
Complementary medicine
Durable medical equipment
Home testing equipment

Services Provided to Specific Populations
Geriatric
Pediatric
Women's health
Disease-specific

Services Associated with a Practice Setting
Hospital
   Centralized services
   Decentralized services
Independent
Chain
Mass merchandiser
Grocery store
Mail order or Internet
Long-term care
Home health

schemes established by service marketers. By fitting their services into these new classifications, pharmacists can explore how providers in similar service categories address parallel situations.

SERVICE CLASSIFICATIONS FROM THE MARKETING FIELD

In this section, classification systems from the general service marketing literature are presented. They are based on variables such as the tangibility of the product–service mix, nature of the service act, and type of provider–customer relationship.

Each of these classification systems attempts to analyze services in ways that offer insight into how the services are provided, how the services may be perceived by consumers, and how new strategies for providing services might be identified. These systems are presented to stimulate pharmacists to think outside the box when analyzing service marketing opportunities. They can provide insights into ways of better serving the customer.

Tangibility of the Product–Service Mix

The service mix provided by pharmacists ranges from product focused to service focused (Figure 3-1). The more product focused the mix is, the more the pharmacist will adopt strategies consistent with the marketing of products. The more service focused the mix is, the more a service strategy is needed.

The left side of Figure 3-1 gives examples of product–service combinations that are more tangible; here, few services are likely to be required in order for the patient to benefit from the product. The right side of the continuum indicates mixes in which intensive services are likely to be needed for the patient to receive a benefit.

The provision of nonprescription (over-the-counter) drugs falls at the left end of the tangibility continuum. Although pharmacists are frequently called upon to assist in the selection of nonprescription drugs, the sale of these products requires few supplemental services beyond delivery and shelf stocking. In fact, nonprescription drugs are common items in vending machines. Home testing kits and other devices require more services, because their use can be more complex than that of nonprescription products. Durable medical equipment, such as crutches and wheelchairs, requires even more service.

Low-service dispensing activities are found to the right of the center of the continuum. Low-service dispensing is defined as the minimal level of prescription services required by law. This type of service is often provided by high-volume, low-cost pharmacies. Further to the right are high-level services—those that involve higher levels of personalized care and may be associated with pharmaceutical care. Services provided in these situations can include therapeutic monitoring, intensive counseling, and screening for medical conditions. Drug information services are at the far right of the continuum.

This continuum can help pharmacists understand the relative product orientation of their businesses. If most of their revenue relies on tangible products such as nonprescription medications and other over-the-counter products, then pharmacists will follow traditional product-oriented marketing strategies. If prescription drugs are the main focus of their business, then a service marketing orientation will be more appropriate.

FIGURE 3-1 Pharmacist services on a continuum of product to service orientation. OTCs = over-the-counter products.

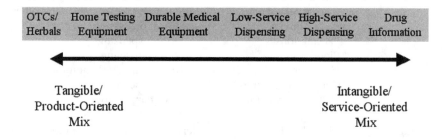

A service marketing orientation requires different strategies than a product orientation does.

Focus of Services

Another way of classifying services is to ask whether they are directed at people or things.[6] Pharmacy services can be classified as (1) tangible actions to people's bodies, such as vaccinations and disease screening; (2) tangible actions to things, such as retail dispensing, veterinary pharmacy, and mail order; (3) intangible actions directed at people, such as patient education and drug information services; or (4) intangible actions directed at intangible assets, such as pharmacy benefit design and drug-use review (Table 3-3).

This categorization is useful because it forces pharmacists to answer some important questions about their services:[6]

1. *Does the patient need to be physically present to receive a pharmaceutical service?* If one considers pharmaceutical services to consist of tangible actions directed at goods, then the answer is probably no. Pharmacists can provide basic dispensing services at a distant location and send the drugs by courier or mail. However, services such as vaccination and cholesterol screening require the presence of the patient.
2. *Does the patient need to be mentally present during the service process?* Intensive counseling sessions require patients to be present, ready, and engaged. If the patient is distracted or fatigued, much of the benefit of counseling will be lost. Services that require mental involvement must be offered whenever and wherever the patient is ready and able to participate. The advantage of the telephone, Internet, and other electronic technologies lies in their ability to provide services at the convenience of the patient.

TABLE 3-3   Pharmacist Services Classified by Nature of the Service Act

Action Type	Directed at People	Directed at Things
Tangible	Services directed at people's bodies Vaccinations Blood pressure monitoring Cholesterol testing Diabetes screening	Services directed at goods and other physical possessions Drug dispensing OTC counseling Durable medical equipment Herbal medicines Veterinary medicine Mail order pharmacy
Intangible	Services directed at people's minds Patient education Drug information services Alternative medicine	Services directed at intangible assets Drug insurance design Pharmacy benefit management Drug-use review

OTC = over-the-counter (nonprescription) product.

Source: Adapted from Reference 2.

This classification system has some limitations. Providers may offer services that fall into more than one category. For example, a pharmacist might give immunizations, a service that clearly falls into the tangible–people category. At the same time, the pharmacist will likely be providing patient education that falls into the intangible–people category. The dispensing of medications is a tangible action directed at a physical good (i.e., a drug), but it also can be considered to be directed at people's bodies. It can be difficult to decide where some services fall.

Type of Pharmacist–Patient Relationship

Pharmacists' services can be classified by the type of relationship with the patient. Relationships can be defined according to (1) whether there is a formal relationship between patient and provider and (2) whether services are provided on a continual basis over time or as discrete transactions.

Many patients have no formal relationship with their pharmacies. Anyone with a prescription can walk into most community pharmacies for service. However, formal relationships are becoming more common. With the advent of drug insurance, customers of prescription drug services often enter into contracts to use network pharmacies. In these relationships, membership is usually with the drug insurance plan, not the pharmacy. In other cases, pharmacy providers develop direct, formal relationships with their customers through loyalty card programs. In loyalty card programs, patients show their card when purchasing merchandise to receive a discount or other benefit. In return, the pharmacy can gather information on patients' purchasing habits and provide incentives to continue patronizing the pharmacy.

Whether pharmacists provide continual or discrete services depends on patient needs and preferences and provider business strategies. If a patient needs to visit a pharmacy only for occasional acute conditions such as a minor skin rash, continual services may be unnecessary. Or, the consumer may prefer to shop at several different pharmacies, depending on price, convenience, or variety. For this consumer, variety and low prices may be more important than continuity. Furthermore, some pharmacies use a high-volume, low-price business strategy that by its very nature can discourage continuity of services. In order to maintain high volume and low prices, patient–pharmacist interactions need to be kept to a minimum, so there is little opportunity to develop a personal relationship. Other pharmacies emphasize a service mix targeted toward patients who desire and need personalized, ongoing care. These providers seek strong bonds with patients who can be served profitably over time.

Room for Customization and Judgment

The role of customization and judgment in the practice of pharmacy has changed over the years. In the past, pharmacists were responsible for compounding most of the drugs provided for customers. They would mix different combinations of medications individualized to each patient's medical condition. Compounding was unique to the pharmacy profession and one of the things that distinguished pharmacists from all other professionals.

Now, pharmacists rarely compound medications in typical practice. Most of the drugs dispensed are purchased from pharmaceutical manufacturers in standardized forms and doses, often in unit-of-use packages (i.e., ready to be dispensed after application of a prescription label). In current practice, most customization by pharmacists comes in the provision of services.

All services can be classified by their potential for customization and judgment.[6] Many services are standardized and do not easily permit customization. For example, people expect that when they enter a movie theater, services will be provided in a set sequence: pay for the ticket, give it to the ticket taker, buy refreshments, find a seat, and see the movie at the scheduled time. Both the service provider and the customer follow this sequence of steps. Most movie theaters serve the same selection of refreshments: popcorn, soft drinks, and candy. This is expected. It is also expected that movie patrons will wait in line, scan the concession menu above the snack bar, and make a choice quickly and without much deviation from the menu.

The provider and customer are expected to act in ways consistent with their roles. If the movie theater makes a substitution for any concession snack item (e.g., fresh vegetables for popcorn), movie patrons may get upset. On the other hand, theater employees will become impatient if a patron orders snack items that are not on the menu. The expectations of both customers and providers discourage the performance of services outside those expectations. Standardized sequences of events occur with mass merchandise retailers, public transportation, quick-oil-change businesses, and many other services.

The potential for customization also depends on the degree to which frontline service personnel can exercise judgment in meeting the needs of customers. In standardized service situations, the responsibilities and roles of customer contact personnel are restricted. A cook in a fast food restaurant is not allowed to provide items that are not on the menu, a bus driver cannot take new routes to a destination, and a quick-oil-change mechanic cannot fix mufflers. In other words, the nature of individual jobs can limit customization.

Jobs such as those in the legal and health care professions cannot be easily standardized. Although some standardization can occur in medicine (e.g., urgent care centers) and law (e.g., standardized wills), many of the problems seen in these professions are too complex for standardized solutions. For instance, problems in surgery and radiation oncology are likely to require solutions that take into account numerous unpredictable factors. Other areas in which standardization is difficult include architecture, home repair, and real estate.

In most businesses the choice between customization and standardization is a strategic decision. Customization can differentiate one business from another and establish a competitive advantage. Customized service can often provide an advantage because it is tailored to the specific needs of customers, but customization can be more expensive because it requires greater personnel time and financial resources. Standardization can lower costs by increasing efficiency so that fewer personnel are needed to serve customers. This can permit businesses to offer lower prices without reducing profitability.

Professional and Nonprofessional Services

Services can be classified as professional or nonprofessional. Professional services are provided by individuals who are members of a profession, such as physicians, lawyers, and pharmacists. Professionals are distinguished from nonprofessionals by the following characteristics:[7]

- Professionals are considered to have unique skills, expertise, and training that nonprofessionals do not.
- Professionals have a distinct group identity and are largely self-regulating.
- Professionals are experts in specialized fields and use their expertise to advise and assist customers in solving problems.

Consumers tend to perceive professional services as important and are inclined to be less sensitive to the pricing of these services.

Professional services are distinct from nonprofessional services in several ways.[7] Professional services are more complex and require more extensive problem-solving skills and expertise. Consumer perceptions of risk are greater with professional services, because of the complexity of problems dealt with by professionals. In addition, consumers perceive themselves to be less able to assess the quality of professional services because of insufficient expertise and training.

Being perceived as a professional has several strategic implications for pharmacists.[7] Consumers tend to perceive professional services as important and are inclined to be less sensitive to the pricing of these services. When professional issues such as health or financial well-being are at stake, consumers are less likely to pinch pennies. Also, perceptions of expertise are more important in selecting professional services. Consumers place greater weight on the technical expertise of professionals because it is this expertise that determines a successful outcome. Finally, word-of-mouth recommendations are more important in marketing communications for professional services than are advertising and other paid forms of promotion. Since professional services are perceived to involve more risk, consumers gravitate toward more credible sources of product and service information, such as recommendations from friends and family.

Nature of Supply and Demand for Services

Services can also be classified according to the nature of supply and demand. Services are perishable, so they cannot be stored for later use. If they are not used immediately once they are produced, they are gone. Thus, an airline seat is wasted if someone does not purchase it by the time the plane takes off. The same is true for a lecture that is skipped by a student pharmacist.

Since services cannot be stored, they are subject to supply and demand imbalances that are not usually seen with manufactured goods. Providers can have downtime in which personnel and resources are available but there are no customers. At other times, there are more customers than can be taken care of with the available personnel and resources.

Service strategies are shaped by the extent to which demand fluctuates over time and the degree to which supply is constrained by the practice setting.[6] Knowing the influence of supply and demand on a business helps marketers understand the limitations they face and suggests new ways of balancing supply and demand. Marketers should consider several important questions about their services.[6]

The first question is, "How predictable are demand variations?" Does customer demand vary according to the time of day, day of the week, week of the month, or month of the year? The predictability of demand depends in part on the customer base being served. The demand of local customers in stable neighborhoods and towns is more predictable than that of transient customer populations such as commuters or people near military bases. Some seasonal demand and periodic demand can be forecasted. Many diseases, such as influenza, allergic rhinitis, and colds, are seasonal. Certain types of infections (e.g., otitis media) are associated with the beginning of daycare and the school year. More employed people tend to visit pharmacies around payday, at lunch, and after work, and Medicaid and Medicare beneficiaries are more likely to visit pharmacies around the dates when they receive their checks.

A second question is, "What are the causes for these demand variations?" There are numerous causes. Many shopping behaviors are based on habit and preferences; most patients are accustomed to being able to visit a pharmacy at any time of the day or week to receive immediate service. Other demand variations are the result of actions by third parties. Patient visits to pharmacies are influenced by physicians (e.g., physician office hours and recommendations) and insurance companies (e.g., through cost control mechanisms such as formulary systems and access controls such as mail order incentives).

A third question is, "Can demand variations be influenced by marketing?" In many cases, the answer is yes. Patients will change their shopping behavior if they are shown that this will reduce their costs or result in better services. Physicians will change their prescribing if they or their patients will benefit. Most physicians readily change a prescription if it is made clear that the patient will save money or be at lower risk for adverse effects. Insurers will change their pharmaceutical benefit controls if they can save money or if patients demand it.

Method of Service Delivery

The final service classification deals with two questions: "Can services be provided from a distance?" and "Should services be offered at a single site or multiple sites?" The answers to these questions can help determine which convenience strategies can be used in providing pharmaceutical services.

Convenience can have different meanings. For some people, convenience means being able to get service at multiple locations within some geographic area (e.g., their town). For others, it means not having to leave one's house or even one's chair to get service.

Convenience may involve tradeoffs. Convenience strategies can lead to problems with quality control. Services that are offered at multiple sites can suffer if not all service personnel receive the same level of training and supervision. It is easier for the owner of a single independent pharmacy to supervise and maintain the quality of pharmacist services than it is for the chief executive officer of a large chain. In addition, service offered by telephone or Internet can hinder communication and understanding, because much communication is nonverbal. Communication by telephone or e-mail has greater potential for misunderstandings and, in the case of pharmacy, treatment failures.

MEETING THE CHALLENGES IN PROVIDING SERVICES

Tangible Clues to Quality

When customers have difficulty evaluating pharmaceutical services because of intangibility, they look for tangible clues to quality. Tangible clues are things such as the lighting, cleanliness, and neatness of a pharmacy practice site. Other tangible clues can include the dress, appearance, and body language of the pharmacist; the manner in which merchandise is organized on the shelves; and the quality of patient information leaflets. Pharmacists who want to project an image of quality must pay attention to these details.

Tangible Evidence of Service

When providing pure services with no tangible product, give people something they can feel and touch as evidence that they have received something of value. When educating patients, give them something in writing, such as a patient package insert or a written care plan, to remind them of what was discussed. In addition to the value provided by the information on the insert or plan, patients then have something to remind them that a valuable transaction took place.

Word-of-Mouth Promotion

The more complex the service, the more likely it is that consumers will use word-of-mouth recommendations from friends, acquaintances, and family members in choosing pharmacists and pharmacies. As personal sources of recommendation become more important, pharmacists should attempt to tap into this trend by encouraging customer "word-of-mouth."

There are several strategies pharmacists can use to increase word-of-mouth communication. The first is to ask customers to recommend the pharmacy to others. The request can be simple: "If you are happy with our service, please recommend us to family or friends." As relationships with customers strengthen, pharmacists should look for opportunities to subtly encourage recommendations. The pharmacist might say, "John, I haven't seen your wife in here lately. Has she been taking her blood pressure medicine consistently?"

Professionalism

Although pharmacy is a profession, not all pharmacists are recognized as professionals by customers. The image of individual pharmacists is determined by how they interact daily with their customers. Pharmacists who consistently demonstrate good decisions, judgment, and professionalism are likely be perceived as professionals. Pharmacists who do not demonstrate their expertise, are unprofessional in their interactions with customers, and minimize patient contact are less likely to be perceived as professionals.

Pharmacists should promote the professional nature of their services. Promotional communications should emphasize pharmacists' expertise, competence, and training. Pharmacists should never pass up an opportunity to teach patients about how they ensure patient safety and positive health outcomes. When a pharmacist identifies a drug-related problem, he should explain to the patient the nature of the problem and the actions he will be taking to resolve it. If every pharmacist did this on a daily basis, people would be more likely to characterize pharmacists as professionals.

Strong Image of the Business

When consumers lack the information or ability to judge the quality of a business, they often rely on general perceptions in choosing where to do business. The greater the perceived risk associated with what the business provides, the more important are general impressions about quality. Many businesses attempt to establish a strong image of their firm in the minds of customers. A well-known and respected image can reduce customers' perception of risk. Think of the names IBM, Microsoft, Mercedes-Benz, and Pfizer. Each evokes a strong image of quality that makes the business stand out from competitors. Similarly, excellent pharmacies and pharmacists can establish and maintain a strong positive image through promotional communications and other elements of the marketing mix.

Relationship Marketing

Pharmacists should target patients who want or need to establish and maintain long-term formal and informal relationships with pharmacists. Pharmacists can benefit in several ways. With formal membership relationships, it is much easier to collect data reflecting the needs and wants of patients. Patients who use loyalty cards or participate in a managed care plan provide identification that can be used to understand purchasing habits. With that information, services can be customized to specific patient needs. Also, membership pricing can be implemented with formal relationships. A single membership fee can be charged for patients who enroll in a disease management or wellness clinic. One price is charged for the bundle of services, rather than separate prices charged a la carte for medication review, physical assessment, counseling, and various other services provided in a program. Finally, patients who maintain long-term formal or informal relationships are cheaper and more profitable to serve. Loyal patients tend to spend more money and be less price-sensitive than other consumers, and they require the same level of advertising and promotion.[8]

Use of Technology

Technology can help pharmacists better serve their patients in several ways. Technologies such as automated telephone routing systems, dispensing robots, computer workflow systems, computer-generated notifications, and computer-assisted inventory management can speed service and free pharmacists from routine clerical tasks. Service quality can be enhanced through electronic prescribing, point-of-service online drug-use review, educational Web pages, electronic patient data systems, and diagnostic technologies such as blood pressure monitors. Access to drugs and services can be made more convenient for patients through telepharmacy and tools such as Internet services, touchscreen interactive kiosks, and ATM-like dispensing machines.

Multiple Sites

The greater the geographic area a pharmacy can cover, the more likely it is that customers will use its services. If customers can visit pharmacy locations near work, at home, and on vacation without changing their pharmacy provider, they will be more likely to establish a relationship with a single pharmacy firm. That is a major reason why large chains have expanded into most geographic areas and have nationwide prescription profile databases that permit pharmacists to refill prescriptions at any pharmacy in the chain, regardless of location.

One of the biggest problems associated with the provision of pharmacy services at multiple sites is quality control. Services at each pharmacy are provided by personnel with different skills, capabilities, attitudes, values, and personalities. Therefore, services can vary substantially from pharmacy to pharmacy. This problem is aggravated by national and regional shortages of qualified pharmacists. Shortages can force pharmacy employers to be less selective in hiring, which can result in greater variations in service. One way of dealing with variations among personnel is to standardize tasks through strict rules and procedures. Another way is to provide extensive employee training and management support.

Storing Services

Although many services are wasted if not consumed immediately after production, others can be saved for use at a later date. Information and educational services can be stored in various media. Books are one of the oldest ways of storing information. Electronic media such as tape recordings, CD-ROMs, and Internet Web pages can expand the capabilities of service providers to store information and educational materials.

Information that is stored can be used when the customer is ready and willing. When a professor presents a lecture, students may be sleepy, distracted by concerns about an upcoming test, or mentally fatigued from learning. But if the main points from the lecture are reinforced in an assigned reading or taped lecture, students can review the information at a later time. Storing information in various media also allows students to choose the form that best fits their style of learning. Some students learn better by reading; others learn better by listening or watching. Another advantage is that, once the information is stored, it can be reproduced to reach many more people. A book can be read by millions of people. An Internet Web site can reach people all over the world.

Storing services for later use presents some challenges. Substantial time and effort are required to store information in a comprehensible and effective form for customers. Even a simple patient education pamphlet can take hours to produce. Good Web pages and books can take thousands of hours to produce. Another challenge is that information changes, and time must be spent updating handouts, Web pages, and other media. Finally, information in print and electronic media lacks the potential for interactivity and involvement that human interaction can provide. Humans can ask questions, interpret information, and respond in a personalized way. Stored information and its presentation are standardized.

Managing Supply and Demand

Pharmacists can do a variety of things to even out the demand for services. One is to encourage customers to visit during nonpeak periods. This can be accomplished by offering discount prices on certain days of the week or coupons that are redeemable only within certain periods. Another way to manage demand is by making people wait for services. Customers who find that it will take the pharmacist an hour to fill their prescription will either take the prescription elsewhere or visit at a different time. Finally, service providers such as pharmacists must make the most of their time during lulls. Paperwork can be completed, calls can be made to physicians and patients, and disease management appointments can be scheduled.

SUMMARY

Most successful businesses attempt to emulate the best practices of all businesses, not just those within their own narrow field. Health care providers now realize that they can learn a lot from the best practices of a variety of service-oriented businesses, including the hospitality, retailing, and food service industries. One of the main goals of this chapter has been to convey the message that the pharmacy profession needs to look beyond its current practices and explore how other businesses serve customers.

References

1. Holdford DA, Yom SH. Content analysis of newspaper advertising of pharmacy services. *J Pharm Mark Manage.* 2003;15(2):81–96.
2. Shostack GL. Breaking free from product marketing. *J Mark.* 1977; 41: 73–80.
3. Gronroos C. *Service Management and Marketing.* Lexington, Mass: Lexington Books; 1990.
4. Zeithaml VA, Parasuraman A, Berry LL. Problems and strategies in services marketing. *J Mark.* 1985;49:33–46.
5. Zeithaml VA, Bitner M. *Services Marketing.* New York: McGraw–Hill Co Inc.; 1996.

6. Lovelock CH. Classifying services to gain strategic marketing insights. *J Mark.* 1983;47:9–20.
7. Hill CJ, Neeley SE. Differences in the consumer decision process for professional vs. generic services. *J Serv Mark.* 1988;2:17–23.
8. Heskett JL, Sasser ED, Schlesinger LA. *The Service Profit Chain.* New York: The Free Press; 1997.

Additional Readings

Hult GT, Lukas BA. Classifying health care offerings to gain strategic marketing insights. *J Serv Mark.* 1995;9(2):36–48.
Parente ST. Beyond the hype: a taxonomy of e-health business models. *Health Aff.* 2000;19(6):89–102.
Vargo SL, Lusch RF. Evolving to a new dominant logic for marketing. *J Mark.* 2004;68(1):1–17.

Exercises and Questions

1. Does the average pharmacy in your community emphasize product-oriented or service-oriented marketing strategies? Explain the reason for your answer.
2. What pharmacist services in your community are primarily directed at people, and what services are directed at things?
3. How might pharmacy services in your community be provided
   a. Through a "membership" relationship?
   b. At a site distant from patients?
   c. In multiple service outlets?
   d. At the home of the customer?
   e. In a standardized manner?
   f. At an interactive, touchscreen kiosk?
4. Are customized or standardized pharmaceutical services better for patients? Explain.
5. Provide arguments for why pharmacist services should be classified as "professional."

Activity

We all have service encounters every week with restaurants, bars, banks, airlines, gas stations, dry cleaners, hair stylists, physicians, libraries, schools, car repair shops, copy centers, and others. Record 10 "journal" entries describing service encounters that you experience in the next week. Attempt to include a variety of service businesses and types (e.g., services provided by automation, over the telephone, by Internet, in person). Include satisfying and dissatisfying encounters. Record factual information (when, where, nature of service encounter), your expectations prior to the encounter, a description of the service delivery process, your assessment of its quality (on a scale from 1 to 10), and your perceptions and feelings about each service experience. Note any concepts from this book that are pertinent to your service experience. It is essential that you complete the journal entries on the day of the service and not rely on your memory to recreate them later. Finally, write a one-page report on what you learned from this experience.

MANAGING SERVICE PERFORMANCE

The pharmacy business today places tremendous emphasis on service. Competition for patients is fierce, and service differentiates one pharmacy from the next. The drugs in any pharmacy are essentially the same, but the service is not. The prescription drug received from a Walgreens store is the same as that filled at CVS. It is the service provided along with the drug that varies from pharmacy to pharmacy. Service can differ in terms of accessibility, merchandise display and selection, professional services, friendliness, helpfulness, and many other dimensions. Service, along with price, determines the success of a pharmacy in gaining and keeping patients.

Not all pharmacies provide good service. I have seen the following examples of poor service in pharmacies:

- All of the other employees laugh as the pharmacist regales them with a story about "telling off" a patient.
- Irritated by the incessant ringing of a telephone, the pharmacist picks up the receiver and slams it back down without answering.
- When a patient complains that the price of a drug is too high, the pharmacist flippantly responds, "You can always go to the pharmacy down the street." A student pharmacist nods his head in agreement.

Situations like these, in which pharmacists give poor service to patients, are not uncommon. Most pharmacists, student pharmacists, and technicians can cite similar instances of poor service. Often they confess that they too have provided poor service at times.

Poor service is not just rude or discourteous behavior. It is failure of pharmacists to meet their professional responsibilities. In a widely publicized study by *U.S. News & World Report*,[1] more than half of 245 pharmacists in seven cities failed to warn consumers who presented prescriptions for drugs with potentially dangerous interactions.

When poor service occurs, it is often because the pharmacist is under stress or because some circumstance causes him or her to act in a way that is not typical. The pharmacist may have been working all day without a break and reacted inappropriately as a result of fatigue and hunger. He or she may have been working without much support from co-workers and management.

But no matter the reason, poor pharmacy service is unacceptable. It cannot be tolerated—by pharmacists, patients, payers, or pharmacy managers. At the very least, poor pharmacy service can cause patients to take their business elsewhere. When patients tell others about their bad service experiences, more business can be lost.

At worst, poor service can cause patient injury or death. Pharmacists who discourage requests for counseling or cut corners by not checking medication profiles can physically harm the people who rely on their professional expertise and behavior. Pharmacists and other health care professionals cannot be permitted the luxury of providing bad service. One lapse in service delivery can destroy years spent building a good patient relationship. It can even end a person's life.

CAUSES OF POOR PHARMACY SERVICE

Some pharmacists do not realize they are providing poor service. A pharmacist who rudely tells the patient, "If you don't like our service, you can go down the street" may not realize that this is unprofessional behavior. We may all feel like expressing our frustrations this way from time to time, but as professionals we must learn to control our impulses. Unfortunately, a pharmacist may learn inappropriate service behavior by observing other, more experienced pharmacists or even a supervisor.

Poor service can also result when a pharmacist is the "wrong fit" for a service job. Not everyone is interested in or suited for working with patients.

On the other hand, some pharmacists who have the potential to provide good service simply have not developed the skills and habits to do so. They may lack sufficient communication and counseling skills or have poor work habits that lead to inefficiency and inattention to detail.

In many cases, poor service is not the fault of the pharmacist but of the system in which the pharmacist works. Poor service can be built into a system through poor design, management, recruitment, retention, and training. For example, failure to screen for drug interactions can have a variety of causes, including computer systems that incorrectly identify potential drug interactions as needing attention, pharmacists who have unclear policies for dealing with drug interactions, and managers who emphasize prescription volume over patient safety. These system problems contribute to poor pharmacist performance.

Providing good customer service is not easy. If it were easy, people would never have their orders mixed up in a restaurant, wait long periods on the telephone or in checkout lines, or be subjected to rude or incompetent service workers.

In the practice of pharmacy, it is particularly difficult to provide good service. Pharmacists are not simply required to provide fast and friendly service. They must maintain accurate patient records, monitor therapy, communicate with and educate patients, and watch out for the patient's welfare.

ELEMENTS OF GOOD CUSTOMER SERVICE

Good customer service depends on several important factors.[2-4] First, it requires the support of a customer-oriented organization—one that emphasizes service leadership, investment in employee training and development, and teamwork. The second key factor is selection and retention of good employees, without whom good service is not possible. Third, good customer service depends on a well-designed and well-run service system. This chapter discusses each of these factors.

Customer-Oriented Organizational Culture

In a customer-oriented organizational culture, everyone recognizes that the organization exists for one reason: to serve the customer.[5,6] People in customer-oriented organizations know that without the customer, there would be no organization. The customer determines the success or failure of the firm. Customer orientation requires that everyone, from the chief executive officer to the service line employee, be devoted to meeting customer needs and wants. Pharmacists are customer oriented if they can respond with an unqualified "yes" to the following statements:

> *Good service organizations have strong leaders who stress the importance of service in both words and actions.*

- I always go out of my way to assist my patients.
- I am never too busy to help co-workers and patients.
- I always persuade patients, rather than pressure them.
- I continually assess my patients' needs.
- I am willing to disagree with patients to help them make better decisions.
- I never put my needs before patients' needs.
- I continually look for opportunities to help my co-workers and patients.
- I never pretend that I cannot help patients and co-workers when I really can.
- I never ignore patients when I am busy.
- I can always control my emotions when dealing with patients and co-workers.

If you answered "yes" to all of these statements, verify the accuracy of your responses by asking trusted co-workers for their assessment of your customer orientation. They may provide a different perspective and offer suggestions for improvement.

Service Leadership

Customer orientation in any pharmacy organization starts at the top. The pharmacy leader sets the organization's direction and priorities. If service is not foremost in the mind of pharmacy leaders, it will not be a priority at the pharmacy staff level.

Good service organizations have strong leaders who stress the importance of service in both words and actions. Such leaders have a strong commitment to service and are able to communicate this to others within the organization. The Ukrop's regional grocery chain provides an example of strong service leadership. Its orientation program for pharmacy department and other store employees includes an introduction to the company's values and commitment to the community by president Bobby Ukrop. All employees, including baggers, cashiers, and stockers, are trained by the president in the importance of serving customers and the community. The emphasis on extraordinary customer service is continually reinforced throughout the company.[7]

Service leadership can occur at many levels. Leadership can be shown by the independent pharmacy owner, the hospital pharmacy director, the chief executive officer of a national pharmacy chain, and even the pharmacist in charge at a community pharmacy. The higher up in an organization the commitment to service exists, the more likely it is that service is an organizationwide priority.

The leader's role in communicating a coherent vision to subordinates cannot be underestimated. A shared vision of service can excite people and motivate them toward common goals.

President John F. Kennedy illustrated the power of vision when he told the world, in the 1960s, that America would have a man on the moon by the end of the decade. At the time, travel to the moon seemed impossible. Nevertheless, President Kennedy's vision helped energize the American people to support the efforts of the U.S. space program. This compelling vision led the nation to put a man on the moon in 1969, after Kennedy's death.

Pharmacy service organizations can benefit from inspirational leadership. The practice of pharmacy is no less important than going to the moon. People put their trust and their health in the hands of pharmacists, and pharmacists should realize that what they do is more than just a job. Practicing pharmacy is too difficult without the feeling that it has some meaning or value. Good leaders can provide pharmacy employees with an inspirational vision of the organization and the profession.

Investment in Training and Development

Excellent pharmacy service organizations invest in the training and development of their employees.[6,8,9] This involves more than just paying pharmacists to attend continuing-education programs to meet state licensing requirements. It means providing job-based training that can help pharmacists to do their jobs better and to progress in their careers.

Pharmacists in service organizations cannot be expected to perform well if they lack the appropriate skills and knowledge to do their jobs correctly. Pharmacists need training and development throughout their careers. Even pharmacists with extensive practice experience need to periodically renew their skills to keep up with changes in the profession.

In addition to updating employees' knowledge, training and development can help build confidence, enhance intrinsic motivation, and promote self-esteem.[6] Often, employees know what to do but lack the confidence or reinforcement to do it. Proper training can provide the impetus to do the right thing for patients even when it is not easy to do so.

Furthermore, training and development enhance service by making daily work more interesting and fulfilling. The more people know about their jobs, the more they can become involved in the details and delivery. A repetitive task, such as filling a prescription, is much more interesting if the pharmacist understands the therapeutics of the drug being dispensed, the diseases suffered by the patient, and the methods and theories of patient counseling. The more the pharmacist knows, the more he or she is enriched by the job.

The most effective training is planned and scheduled, and the methods are based on the needs of the individual and the organization. Some skills might be learned from another employee, others might be developed through a continuing-education program offered by a pharmacy association, and others might be learned on the job through trial and error. Whatever the training method, the goal should be to help pharmacists and other employees serve customers better.

Teamwork

The practice of pharmacy can be demanding and stressful, and pharmacists need the support of co-workers. Pharmacists' workload often is heavy, and without assistance they cannot practice pharmacy the way they would like to. A community pharmacist may have one patient who requires extensive counseling about a medication, another who wants to discuss why his insurance company will not pay for his medication, a third who has a potential drug interaction, and three more patients who need their prescriptions filled. If not working as part of a team, the pharmacist will find it impossible to satisfy all of these patients.

Teamwork enables pharmacists to meet the demands of their jobs. Knowing that other pharmacists and technicians are available and willing to help can reduce stress when things get busy. In addition to helping with the physical work, co-workers can offer moral support. For instance, a pharmacist who has just been criticized by a physician or patient may be quite upset. Co-workers can help by simply listening while the pharmacist vents frustrations and concerns.

Co-workers can also share successful solutions to problems. In some pharmacies, unusual or difficult problems are documented in a notebook that is reviewed periodically by all employees. The employee involved writes a description of the problem, the circumstances surrounding it, and how it was solved. Another way employees can benefit from the experiences of others is through periodic meetings to discuss interesting patient cases. One pharmacist describes a difficult patient case and how he or she dealt with it, and learning takes place through group discussion.

Often, pharmacists work with nonpharmacist professionals on interdisciplinary teams. A specific problem (e.g., how do we reduce medication errors?) may be identified and addressed in team meetings. Since many problems and solutions in pharmacy practice originate outside the pharmacy organization, participation on interdisciplinary teams is important.

Selecting and Keeping Good Employees

Quality service is built through the selection and retention of quality workers. Employers compete for talented pharmacy employees, not just to fill open positions but to keep good employees from leaving to work for competitors.

Excellent service organizations try hard to recruit excellent workers. The best service workers have not only good skills and intelligence, but the right attitude. Employers select and keep service employees who have a good balance of knowledge, skills, and attitude. Characteristics of excellent service employees are listed in Table 4-1.

Internal Marketing

Employers need to market themselves to attract and keep talented employees; this is internal marketing.[11] Employers have a product (i.e., a job) that needs to be marketed to customers (i.e., potential and current employees). Some components of the product are a good work environment, acceptable pay and benefits, and the opportunity to learn and progress within the job.

Employers can aggressively market to potential and existing employees. In internal marketing, management treats employees the same way external customers are treated. Employers conduct market research to identify employee needs (e.g., through employee satisfaction surveys), develop an attractive product offering (e.g., salary, challenging work), and promote that offering through different forms of marketing communication (e.g., want ads, word of mouth).

TABLE 4-1 Characteristics of Excellent Service Employees

Service Attitude
It is very important to hire people with the right attitude; skills can be taught. Good customer service requires people who are motivated to help customers. Some people enjoy service jobs. Others, although equally talented, are not right for service positions. It is important to find people with the right fit.

Natural Intelligence
This refers to the mental capabilities of employees to analyze and solve problems. The level of natural intelligence that employees need depends on the type of work they do. The more they are required to deal with complex rather than routine problems, the more natural intelligence they need.

Technical Skills
This refers to the knowledge and experience required to do a job. In general, pharmacists need knowledge about drugs, an understanding of the disease process, and familiarity with organizational rules, regulations, and procedures. Technical skills are highly job dependent; for example, a staff pharmacist needs greater technical knowledge of drugs and diseases, while managers have more need to understand rules, regulations, and procedures.

Emotional Intelligence
This refers to the "people skills" associated with a job. Emotional intelligence comes with maturity and life experience and is considered the most important factor in a person's success or failure on the job.[10] It involves the following:

1. Self-knowledge: An understanding of one's emotions, weaknesses, and bad habits
2. Self-control: The ability to control one's emotions, weaknesses, and bad habits
3. Personal motivation: The ability to maintain one's motivation for a task through good times and adversity
4. Empathy: The ability to understand and be sensitive to another's emotions and differences
5. Ability to influence change: The ability to persuade others to accept new ideas

The more desirable the job, the better management is able to select the best employees to serve customers. An employer that has and markets the best jobs becomes the employer of choice for employees. Employers of choice have fewer problems with job turnover, because employees do not want to leave. When vacancies occur, they are filled quickly. In many cases, want ads are unnecessary; word-of-mouth recommendations from current employees result in a sufficient number of applicants.

Internal marketing to employees has been linked to both satisfaction of external customers[12] and profitability.[13] The relationships among internal marketing, customer service, and profitability of the firm can be

FIGURE 4-1 The service–profit cycle. (Compiled from reference 8.)

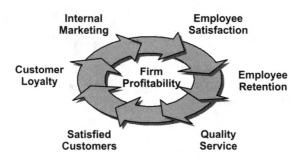

envisioned as a continuous cycle (Figure 4-1).[8] Treating employees well leads to employee satisfaction and retention. Satisfied employees are more likely to appreciate their jobs and have the attitude necessary to provide good service. Happy employees project that happiness to customers and are more enjoyable to be around. Customers are more satisfied and likely to be loyal. Loyal customers generate greater revenue and greater profit for the firm.

The development of an internal marketing environment involves the following steps:[14]

■ Educating employees about the internal marketing concept and the existence of internal customers.
■ Having employees and managers identify their internal customers.
■ Helping employees and managers identify the expectations of their internal customers.
■ Developing strategies to meet the needs of internal customers, such as providing opportunities for professional development and job enrichment for subordinates.
■ Monitoring internal customer satisfaction and other benchmark measures (e.g., customer satisfaction surveys, exit interviews, employee telephone hotlines, suggestion boxes).

Employee Recruitment

Excellent service employers never stop searching for employees. Even when no positions are open, they keep a list of potential employees whom they can contact when an opening occurs. They proactively develop a pool of qualified candidates through work contacts and networking at professional meetings. Current employees also help by recommending the company to potential candidates and contacting them when a position opens.

Proactive recruitment is useful because little time is lost when employees leave. When an opening occurs, qualified candidates are interviewed and hired as quickly as possible in order to maintain continuity of service. This puts them one step ahead of reactive organizations that start recruiting only when a job opening occurs.

> *Pharmacists build bonds of trust with their patients, and those bonds are extended to the pharmacy.*

Employee Retention

Keeping good employees is one of the biggest challenges faced by pharmacist employers. The loss of key employees can have a devastating effect on pharmacies. In one neighborhood in Virginia, people still talk about "Billy," a pharmacist at a pharmacy chain store. Billy lived in the neighborhood of the pharmacy, and many people who visited the pharmacy were his friends. After he left, the store was never the same. Temporary pharmacists rotated in and out. Patients lost their sense of loyalty to the store and started going to nearby competitors. Even years after Billy's departure, patients complained that they missed the relationship they'd had when he was their pharmacist.

Pharmacists build bonds of trust with their patients, and those bonds are extended to the pharmacy. When a key pharmacist leaves, the bond to both the employee and the pharmacy is broken. A new pharmacist has to rebuild the bond, and that can take time.

The cost of losing a pharmacist can be high. The costs of replacing a staff employee in the average business (e.g., costs for recruitment, selection, and training) are $1,000–$2,000 for service workers and $4,000–$8,000 for professionals.[14,15] These numbers do not include costs such as managerial time, lost efficiency, productivity losses, and lost business associated with new employees. One author calculated this cost to be as much as $100,000 for professional and managerial employees.[16]

The loss of a pharmacist can cause multiple problems:

- The pharmacy may have to reduce store hours until a replacement can be found.
- Patients may go to competitors.
- The remaining pharmacists and employees have to cover the responsibilities of the missing pharmacist. This can increase employee stress and lead to more overtime costs to the pharmacy.

- The employer incurs costs to replace the pharmacist. The employer may pay to advertise the position in newspaper want ads or professional journals. Current personnel must be paid for performing related clerical and interviewing tasks.
- Personnel need to be freed from their usual responsibilities so they can train newly hired pharmacists.
- A new pharmacist may take a year or more to become 100% productive. Productivity is reduced while the pharmacist learns job details such as the location of drugs, computer system procedures, and proper handling of insurance forms.

Employers need to invest as much in keeping employees as they do in recruiting them. Adopting an internal marketing philosophy is a good start. In pharmacy practice, excellent service comes down to finding and keeping excellent workers. Without excellent employees, it is much more difficult to succeed in marketing.

Well-Designed and Well-Run Service Systems

Even the best employees have difficulty providing good service in service settings that are poorly designed and run. In many businesses, poor service is designed into the system, as illustrated in the following scenarios.

Scenario 1: At 8:55 am, a hospital nurse goes to the medication room to get a 9 am medication for a patient but finds no drug in the patient's cassette. Knowing how much work she has to do, the nurse tries to save time by checking the medication cassettes of other patients for an extra dose that she can "borrow." Having no luck, she telephones the pharmacy. A pharmacist answers after the 15th ring. The nurse asks the pharmacist to send the missing medication to the nursing unit as soon as possible. The pharmacist checks the patient's computer record to see if an order has been received for the medication. Finding no record of the order in the computer, the pharmacist asks the nurse to see if the order has been sent to the pharmacy yet. Exasperated, the nurse hangs up the phone and searches for the order on the nursing unit. She quickly finds that the order has not yet been picked up by the hospital courier. Knowing that the patient needs the dose before a scheduled X-ray procedure at 10 am, the nurse goes to the central pharmacy to have the medication order filled. At the central pharmacy, she has to wait for 5 minutes while the pharmacy staff assists other nurses. When it is her turn, the nurse receives the medication and returns to the floor. The dose is administered at 9:25 am, and the nurse spends the rest of the day trying to make up the lost 30 minutes.

This situation occurs thousands of times daily in hospitals around the United States. Neither the nurse nor the pharmacist is at fault here. Both are doing their best to provide excellent care to patients. Nevertheless, the nurse has just wasted 30

> *Only when quality is defined and measured will service providers make it a priority.*

minutes on a problem that was preventable. The nurse and the pharmacist are working in a system in which problems like the missing medication are inevitable. The problems are built into the system.

> *Scenario 2:* At 8:55 am, a hospital nurse goes to the medication room to get a 9 am dose and finds it in the patient's cassette. The pharmacist, who is located on the nursing unit, has already picked up the order, keyed it into the computer, and placed the medication in the patient's cassette. The nurse gives the medication to the patient at 8:57 am.

In scenario 2, the pharmacist is better located to serve the nurse. A system is in place that permits the pharmacist to quickly receive and fill new orders. The pharmacist can consult with nurses and physicians face-to-face if any questions arise. In addition, the pharmacist is able to develop better professional relationships with nurses and physicians. This can help reduce conflict and misunderstandings. The service in scenario 2 is better because the system is better. Chapter 5, Designing Pharmacy Services, discusses this topic in more detail.

Quality Improvement

All well-run service organizations have some form of quality improvement (QI) program. Such programs may be called total quality management, continuous quality improvement, six-sigma, or other names, but they share several underlying principles:

- Improvement must be continuous. The assumption is that the status quo is not sufficient for survival in the marketplace. Quality that is adequate now will not be enough in the near future. Quality can be enhanced by continually simplifying the service process, eliminating duplication and unnecessary actions, decreasing process time, and preventing errors.
- Quality must be customer centered. All improvements must be recognized and valued by customers. Quality from the provider's viewpoint is relevant only in relationship to the desires of customers.
- Quality must be measured. This idea is expressed in the maxims "If it is not measured, it is not important" and "Only that which is measured gets accomplished." Only when quality is defined and measured will service providers make it a priority. And only then will providers be able to assess quality and improve it.

FIGURE 4-2 Steps in quality improvement.

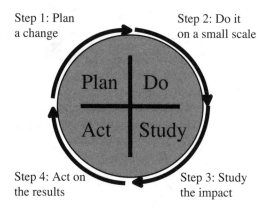

Step 1: Plan
a change

Step 2: Do it
on a small scale

Step 4: Act on
the results

Step 3: Study
the impact

- Solutions to problems should be multidisciplinary. Most quality deficiencies are not located within a single discipline or department. A medication error by a patient can be caused by actions of the pharmacist, technician, physician, or insurer. Solutions to quality problems must cross organizational and professional lines.
- Mistakes are part of the service system. Poorly designed systems set individuals up to make mistakes through overwork, inadequate training or tools to do the job, or myriad other causes. Quality indicators should be used to find and fix problems in the system that result in poor quality, not to punish people who make errors. People who make mistakes are not bad, only human.

Figure 4-2 depicts four steps in QI: Plan, Do, Study, and Act.

Plan. Service providers plan a service improvement by consulting everyone involved in the process. In pharmacy, this might include technicians, nurses, managers, and physicians. These individuals discuss common and important problems in the system that hinder their ability to serve patients. The purpose is to identify problems to target for QI interventions.

Once a problem is targeted, baseline quality indicators are identified and collected to compare with postimprovement measures. For instance, wait times for filling new prescriptions might be targeted because of patient and pharmacist complaints. The indicator, time from dropping off the prescription to picking it up, could be measured before and after any intervention. The QI team could use data on wait time averages and ranges to develop new improvement strategies and adjust old ones.

Ideally, indicators should originate from data already being collected, such as sales figures, customer complaint records, or employee surveys.

FIGURE 4-3 Common quality improvement tools.

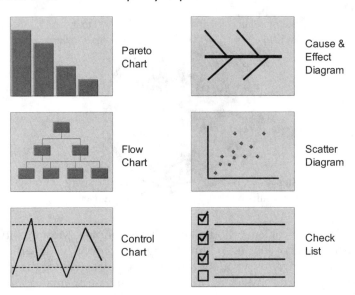

The more difficult it is to collect quality indicators, the less likely it is that they will be gathered. It is helpful for everyone involved to have a basic understanding of statistical quality control techniques.

Do. Once a problem is identified for improvement, an action plan is developed and put into place. Action to reduce dispensing errors might involve the use of a new double-check system before any prescription is dispensed. QI strategies typically are initiated on a small scale so that any problems identified during implementation can be more easily resolved.

Study. After the intervention, data are collected for analysis of the success and unintentional consequences of the effort. The data might be studied to see if the action plan was implemented as decided, to identify correctable flaws in planning and implementation, or to identify new problems within the system that require intervention.

QI tools such as those in Figure 4-3 facilitate the analysis. For instance, a Pareto chart might be used to display the total number of dispensing errors in order of frequency of their causes. A discovery that errors after the QI intervention are more frequently due to pharmacist interruptions might suggest a direction for future QI interventions.

Act. At this point, the entire process of monitoring and assessment starts over again. The purpose is to continually seek out problems within the system and resolve them. This approach reduces errors, waste, inefficiencies, and the costs of serving customers.

In any service system, feedback and accountability are essential. Most managers and employees know that "If it is not measured, it is not important." When the quality of service is never systematically measured or assessed, there is little pressure to improve. QI makes assessment and improvement part of everyday practice.

SUMMARY

Good pharmacy services do not just happen. They require much effort on the part of leaders, managers, and pharmacists. Leaders set forth a vision of excellent services. Managers make certain that vision is followed through actions such as recruitment, training, and internal marketing. Pharmacists provide good services day in and day out by working hard, paying attention to detail, and staying alert for ways to meet the needs of patients.

References

1. Headden S, Lenzy R, Kostyu P, et al. Danger in the drugstore: too many pharmacists fail to protect consumers against potentially hazardous interactions with prescription drugs. *US News World Rep.* August 26, 1996; 46–51, 53.
2. Craig S, Crane VS, Hayman JN, et al. Developing a service excellence system for ambulatory care pharmacy services. *Am J Health Syst Pharm.* 2001; 58:1597–606.
3. Horwitz FM, Neville MA. Organization design for service excellence: a review of the literature. *Hum Resour Manage.* 1996;35:471–92.
4. Redman T, Mathews BP. Service quality and human resource management. *Pers Rev.* 1998;27:47–77.
5. Berry L, Conant JS, Parasuraman A. A framework for conducting a services marketing audit. *J Acad Market Sci.* 1991;19:255–68.
6. Zeithaml VA, Bitner M. *Services Marketing.* New York: McGraw-Hill Co Inc; 1996.
7. Miller CW. Ukrop's service, commitment starts at the top. *Roanoke Times.* April 1, 2001.
8. Heskett JL, Jones TO, Loveman GW, et al. Putting the service-profit chain to work. *Harv Bus Rev.* 1994;72:164–74.
9. Hoffman KD, Bateson JEG. *Essentials of Services Marketing.* Orlando, Fla: Harcourt College Publishers; 2002.
10. Goleman D. What makes a leader? *Harv Bus Rev.* November–December 1998:93–102.
11. Sasser ED, Arbeit SP. Selling jobs in the service sector. *Bus Horiz.* 1976; 19: 61–7.
12. Gremler DD, Bitner MJ, Evans KR. The internal service encounter. *Logist Inf Manage.* 1995;8:28–34.
13. Schlesinger LA, Heskett JL. The service-driven service company. *Harv Bus Rev.* 1991;69:71–81.

14. Reynoso J, Moores B. Towards the measurement of internal service quality. *Int J Serv Ind Manage.* 1995;6:64–83.
15. Weinberg CR, Brushley CD. Stop the job hop! *Chief Exec.* 1997;122:44–7.
16. Fitz-Enz J. It's costly to lose good employees. *Workforce.* 1997;76:51–2.

Additional Readings

Jackson TL. Application of quality assurance principles: teaching medication error reduction skills in a "real world" environment. *Am J Pharm Educ.* 2004;68(1):1–12. Article 17.
Kelly WN, Rucker TD. Compelling features of a safe medication-use system. *Am J Health Syst Pharm.* 2006;63:1461–8.
Saxe R, Weitz BA. The SOCO scale: a measure of the customer orientation of salespeople. *J Mark Res.* 1982;19:343.

Exercises and Questions

1. From your experiences, what do you think is the greatest cause for poor pharmacist service?
2. Discuss the role of pharmacist appearance in patient perceptions of service.
3. Relate the concept of the four I's of intangibility, inconsistency, inventory, and inseparability to the importance of selecting pharmacy personnel.
4. Why might a pharmacy benefit from practicing internal marketing with its employees?
5. What barriers to providing the best possible service do the pharmacists in your practice setting face? Compare your answer with issues discussed in this chapter.

Activities

1. Read the mission statement of your pharmacy. How does it emphasize service to customers? Do you receive messages consistent with this mission from your boss and the other managers with whom you interact?
2. Ask 20 people to describe an instance in which they received especially bad service from a business. Group the responses into common categories of your choosing (e.g., a promise not kept). Organize the responses into a bar chart that shows the primary cause of poor service.

CHAPTER 5

DESIGNING PHARMACY SERVICES

After studying this chapter, the reader should be able to

❏ Compare and contrast the production line approach and the empowerment approach to designing and managing pharmacy services.
❏ Explain the concept of service scripts and their value in providing excellent pharmacy services.
❏ List the steps involved in service recovery.
❏ Discuss the purpose of a service blueprint. Identify the key components and the steps involved in building the blueprint.
❏ Describe the main elements of a service audit. Give examples of questions associated with each element.

In the following scenario,[1] a physician describes his experience as a user of health care services.

"I have chronic microscopic hematuria, and my new primary care physician suggested I have a follow-up intravenous pyelogram (IVP). 'Simple enough,' I thought. She authorized the IVP at a local, well-known medical center and told me to schedule the appointment myself. Thus, the saga began.

"The prominent Yellow Pages advertisement for this renowned institution listed many numbers, none of which seemed correct. I therefore called the main hospital number and was greeted by a recording, informing me that I had called a world-class medical center. The same message was then repeated in Spanish, and the electronic receptionist asked me twice, once in Spanish and once in English, in what language I wanted the rest of the message. I chose English and was given options I could choose by telephone. None of these seemed appropriate, and so I pressed the button connecting me, at last, to a live operator....

"When I reached a live operator, I asked to schedule an IVP. The answer was, 'What's that?' Luckily, I could explain that an IVP is an outpatient x-ray examination of my kidneys. She transferred me to another line. After 13 unanswered rings, I hung up....

"My [first contact with the medical center] left me aggravated and frustrated. Six months passed before guilt and anxiety led me to schedule the IVP. I knew the ropes and was able to navigate more quickly the phone system to the radiology scheduling line, this time answered promptly. I asked for an appointment for my IVP and was told, 'Patients cannot schedule their own exams.' I protested but to no avail. The 'proper procedure' was for my doctor's office to schedule the exam. When I suggested that my doctor had no information whatsoever about my schedule, I was greeted by a silence strongly implying, 'So what?'...

"So, I called my physician's office. The receptionist could not schedule my IVP; it was necessary for me to talk to my doctor, only available to take calls between 1 and 2 PM. I eventually made the call, and after waiting at a pay phone on hold for 5 minutes, I reached my physician. She was most accommodating. I gave her several dates, and she told me she would get back to me. At home a message was waiting, giving me a date 2 weeks in the future. I was instructed to return to her office and pick up my new authorization, which I did by making a special trip several days later....

"The day of the exam arrived. My wife drove me to the medical center, but we misread our city map and arrived 10 minutes late. No signs at the hospital directed us to parking for outpatient services, although the sign for valet parking was clearly in view. I made a stab at going through the emergency entrance, while my wife found a place to park. I found no sign to lead me to an information desk, but I wandered to an appropriate-appearing desk, where a very pleasant woman promptly directed me to the elevators that led to the IVP suite. I arrived at the unit, which was clearly marked in large letters: Mammography....

"I apologized to the receptionist for being late and putting her unit off schedule. She told me, very pleasantly, not to worry. 'Just give me your blue card,' she said, 'and we'll get you started.' 'What blue card?' 'Oh, your registration card.' 'I don't have one.' 'You need to get one.' My heart sank. I tried [to resolve the problem by asking,] 'Why not do my exam first, so that you (and I) can keep to our schedule? I'll register afterward.' The receptionist answered pleasantly but firmly, 'I can't do that. Take 2 long lefts down this corridor, go up to the second floor, turn right, and you will be at registration.' I suspected she had done this before....

"Off I went. I was able to follow her directions, even though there was no signage to direct me to the registration desk. The clerk at the registration desk seemed to regard me as an interruption. She continued to carry on a conversation with her counterpart behind her, ignoring me except to ask a question. I did get my blue card. My name was misspelled....

The design and management of pharmacy organizations determine the quality of services provided.

"Back to the mammography unit for my IVP. I watched as, in the next 10 minutes, with unfailing patience and courtesy, the receptionist gave directions to 4 patients who had arrived at the wrong place.

"The radiology tech escorted me to my exam room, 50 minutes late. The technician, nurse, and radiology resident were pleasant and supportive. No one seemed concerned about the delay. When I commented about late starts, the nurse said, 'If you think you're late, wait until they finish the 22 cardiac caths they have scheduled today.' The procedure went very smoothly. On my way out, I stopped to compliment the receptionist for her patience and persistently good customer service. She beamed, 'You don't know how nice it is to hear that.'"

Source: Adapted with permission from the *Journal of the American Medical Association*. Kenagy JW, Berwick DM, Shore MF. Service quality in health care. *JAMA*. 1999;281:661–5. Copyrighted 1999, American Medical Association.

Events like these are all too common. The patient who goes to the hospital for a relatively simple procedure encounters poor service. And, though we might think that a patient who is a physician would be able to avoid most of the problems an average health care consumer might face, that was not the case here.

Many of the problems in this scenario are designed into the system. Most likely the employees are hard workers who want to help patients, but their hands are tied by poorly designed systems and inflexible policies and procedures. The same problems can be seen in the provision of pharmacy services. The design and management of pharmacy organizations determine the quality of services provided. Pharmacies that are well run can meet the needs of customers effectively and efficiently. Poorly run pharmacies cost more to operate and are less effective in serving patients. Chase and Hayes[2] categorized the quality of service organizations as follows:

Available for service. Organizations that fall into this category look at services as necessary evils. Services are not an important part of the business strategy and are considered only as an afterthought. Management provides minimal support for service operations. Service employees are considered an expense to the organization, not an asset. The primary message from management regarding services is "Don't screw up."

Journeyman. Organizations in this category realize that they must provide services in order to compete. However, service is provided more in response to competitors than in response to customer needs. In other words, the goal is to make services minimally competitive. Over time, these organizations begin to resemble their competitors. As in the previous category, employees are considered an expense to the organization, not an asset.

Distinctive competence. Organizations in this category have a customer focus and continually work to meet customer needs. Service is an integral part of organizational strategy, and resources are committed to providing excellent service. Employees are considered assets to the firm, because they are important in attracting and keeping customers. Customers recognize that the service is different from that of competitors.

World-class service delivery. Organizations in this category are considered not only excellent but innovative. Employees are treated as assets because they generate revenue and are a source of innovations. At the same time, employee performance standards are very demanding. World-class service companies set the standard for all others.

Most likely, there are pharmacy organizations in each of these categories, although few can survive for long in the first two categories. This chapter describes how pharmacy organizations can design and manage services in ways that help the organization stand out from competitors.

APPROACHES TO SERVICE DESIGN

Two broad approaches can be taken to the design and management of excellent service.[3] The production line approach attempts to standardize service performance, simplify tasks, and keep decision-making authority in the hands of management. In contrast, the empowerment approach encourages employees to take greater responsibility for their jobs and to exercise initiative in performing them. This approach attempts to motivate employees to act independently to give excellent, individualized service to each customer.

Production Line Approach

The production line approach is based on the philosophy that customers' needs can best be met with services that are efficient, low cost, and consistent. In production line organizations, management designs the service system, and employees provide the services exactly as designed. A top-down approach is used, and employees are required to act as cogs in a smoothly running service machine. Management's goals are to standardize service performance, simplify tasks, provide a clear division of labor, substitute equipment and systems for employees when possible, and minimize the need for employees to make independent decisions.[4,5]

McDonald's is a well-known example of production line organization in the fast food business. The McDonald's strategy is to make every restaurant in the chain provide the same high-quality food and service. The service employees typically are low-wage, low-skilled workers who are trained to do exactly what they are taught in cooking the food and serving the customers. Each employee has a simple, clearly defined task that is to be done quickly and efficiently. When possible, technology is used to simplify the task and replace employees. Independent decisions by employees (e.g., offering to place blue cheese on a cheeseburger, giving a free meal to good customers) are discouraged.

Production line approaches can be found in high-prescription-volume pharmacies such as mail order pharmacies.[6,7] Dispensing tasks are standardized and simplified as much as possible. The responsibilities of pharmacists and technicians are clearly divided, with technicians attempting to free up the pharmacists for more complex tasks. When possible, robots, automated telephone systems, Internet services, dispensing machines, computers, and other technology are substituted for employees. Staffing is kept to a minimum, so little time may be available for pharmacists to make professional decisions or provide individualized services to patients.

In production line pharmacies, efficiency is demanded of employees.[6,7] Service is defined in terms of speed and accuracy of dispensing. The greater the efficiency, the lower is the personnel cost per prescription dispensed. An additional benefit of the production line approach is that tasks are simplified so that employees can be quickly trained and easily replaced if they quit. In pharmacy chains that use the production line approach, simplification and standardization permit employees to be moved from pharmacy to pharmacy, depending on the immediate need. Managers can use pharmacists and technicians as interchangeable parts of the service system.

Empowerment Approach

The nature of services (i.e., intangibility, simultaneous consumption and production, heterogeneity, perishability) has caused many managers and scholars to argue that service workers should be given significant discretion in how they deal with customers.[8-11] They argue that the interactive nature of services requires that workers be permitted to make prompt and independent decisions to meet each customer's needs. If workers are given the authority and resources, they can identify and correct potential problems before they happen, correct service failures once they occur, and be responsive to the dynamics of service situations.

Empowerment is the term commonly used for giving employees increased authority and flexibility in how they do their jobs. Definitions of empowerment vary, but most agree that empowerment means employees are permitted to exercise some degree of discretion in the delivery of services.[9] Instead of limiting employee actions with strict policies and procedures for the correct way to serve customers, employees are given discretion in how to best serve customers.

Compared with the production line approach, empowered employees have greater responsibility in the provision of service. Empowered employees do not say, "It's not my job" when customer problems occur. They take charge of resolving problems and finding ways to prevent future difficulties.

The empowerment approach assumes that frontline service workers know more than management does about serving individual customers. Therefore, workers are freed from unnecessary rules and regulations that constrain their ability to act in the customer's best interest. One problem with rigid policies and procedures is that they can reduce employee risk taking, leading employees to use policies as an excuse for not helping customers. Most people have faced a service employee who says "It's against our policy" in response to some simple request. In that organization, management has established an environment in which it is probably easier and safer for the employee to tell a customer no rather than risk breaking a policy. Doing the right thing for a customer is often riskier than blindly adhering to inflexible rules.

Excellent service organizations empower their employees to do what is necessary to serve the customer, without substantial constraints. At one department store renowned for its service, the employee handbook gives the following directions for dealing with customers: "Rule 1: Use your good judgment in all situations. There are no additional rules." This is a strong statement by management that employees are empowered to decide

TABLE 5-1   Benefits and Costs of the Empowerment Approach

Benefits	Costs
Better ability to respond to the unique needs of customers	Slower service
	Potentially higher labor costs
More individualized service	Employees cannot be easily interchanged
Better ability to quickly resolve problems	Less easy to replace employees with part-timers
Greater sense of employee ownership about their jobs	Technology is less able to replace empowered employees, because their output is less standardized (for technology to be used, standardization of tasks is necessary)
Greater sense of responsibility for service and outcomes	
Lower turnover, absenteeism, presence of trade unions	
Greater employee warmth and enthusiasm in customer interactions	Greater need for flexible leadership
Intrapreneurism by employees	Employers have to be willing to accept that empowered employees will sometimes make bad decisions
Word of mouth and customer loyalty	

Source: Reference 3.

how to best serve customers, rather than consult management about what is appropriate.

Benefits of Empowerment

Table 5-1 lists benefits of the empowerment approach. One of the main benefits is that employees can provide individualized services in response to the unique needs of customers. In each service situation, there are "moments of truth" in which a customer can be gained or lost. The empowerment approach permits employees to respond quickly to opportunities to provide excellent service and solve problems resulting from poor service. Decisions do not need to be made through the manager.

It is hard for managers to encourage exceptional services through policies and procedures, because policies and procedures cannot address all service situations. Instead, exceptional services are accomplished because frontline employees want to serve their customers and are able to do so. The following conditions tend to be associated with exceptional services.[12]

Adaptability of employees. Adaptability refers to the flexibility of employees in responding to customer needs and requests. Customers appreciate it when service providers expend extra effort to adapt to special needs or requests. This differs from situations in which providers quote rules that limit their ability to provide anything beyond the norm. Sometimes, being adaptable even means breaking the rules. For example, it may be necessary for a pharmacist to dispense an emergency drug without all of the necessary documentation. It may break the rules, but in some situations it can be the most appropriate course of action.

Spontaneity of employee actions. Customers often appreciate unprompted and unsolicited employee actions, such as an offer to deliver medication to a patient's home or help choose a nonprescription cold medicine. Customers remember spontaneous actions by employees that result in special attention or some other bonus.

An employee's ability to cope. Employees who can handle difficult situations without losing their composure (i.e., demonstrate grace under pressure) are associated with exceptional services. Snapping at co-workers or patients when the workload gets heavy reveals poor coping skills. Pharmacists with good coping skills maintain their composure no matter how heavy the workload.

Recovery. Recovery refers to an employee's response to a failure in service delivery. The response after making a dispensing error, running out of a drug, or not meeting a promise is one of the most critical factors in determining whether a customer remains loyal to a service provider.[12–14] When a pharmacist or pharmacy makes a mistake, the response can help recover any respect, confidence, or faith that has been lost.

Empowerment can make employees feel better about their jobs.[9] Empowerment by management demonstrates respect for employees. It says that management trusts the capabilities of employees enough to share responsibility with them and treat them as valued adults. Empowerment also increases feelings of ownership; this results in better feelings about the job itself. Think about how people differ in their treatment of a house they rent and one they own. With ownership, people take greater pride in their home and spend more time on maintenance and repair. The same is true about job ownership. Employees who feel ownership of a job take greater interest in what they do and how well it is done. Ownership enhances employee feelings about the job because it increases the perception that the employee's work has meaning. Employees who feel good about their jobs show greater warmth and enthusiasm when they interact with customers.

Costs of Empowerment

Table 5-1 also lists costs of the empowerment approach. Empowerment requires more leadership from management. Rather than directing employees to accomplish tasks, managers need to inspire employees to take responsibility for the job. This can be difficult for managers who are used to working in a production line system. It requires managers to be teachers, coaches, and team leaders.

Managers also need to change employee attitudes about work. Many employees have never had to accept responsibility for their work. Employees must realize that they will be held accountable for more than just showing up. They need to understand that their performance and rewards will be assessed against measures of group output. For example, pharmacist and technician performance may be evaluated with measures such as pharmacy profitability, number of repeat customers, and sales volume.

Employees need sufficient information about their jobs if they are to share responsibility with management.[3,9] They need information that will help them appreciate where their job fits within the overall context of the organization, because many service decisions depend on understanding the consequences of different courses of action. For example, a pharmacist who does not charge a patient for a prescription needs to understand the financial impact that will have on the organization.

Another cost of the empowerment approach is that it is often less efficient and can result in service that is slower and more expensive. In production line organizations, labor costs per unit of output tend to be lower. The following statistics illustrate some of the efficiencies associated with a production line mail order pharmacy at a Department of Veterans Affairs facility:[6]

- Each full-time-equivalent staff member can fill 50,000 to 75,000 prescriptions per year, compared with 8,000 to 18,000 per year in more traditional pharmacies.
- Each pharmacist checks up to 1,000 prescriptions for accuracy during an average 8-hour shift.
- The accuracy of prescriptions dispensed was 99.989% in 1997. Newer systems are able to increase this rate even further.
- Nondrug costs for each prescription dispensed in 1997 were approximately $2.12, including personnel, overhead, and mailing costs. Cost-of-dispensing studies for community pharmacies frequently put nondrug costs at more than twice that amount.[15]

Finally, empowered employees can make bad decisions. It is possible to go too far in pleasing customers. For example, a pharmacist may decide to solve a conflict by offering to give the customer a $50 prescription at no charge. With loyal customers, it may be good business sense to generate goodwill that results in future revenue. But the $50 can be a significant portion of the day's profit for the pharmacy and may never result in any customer goodwill.

Which Approach Is Better?

Most pharmacies use a combination of the empowerment and production line approaches to provide service. Even the most empowered employees need structure in their jobs. On the other hand, it is impossible to control every aspect of employee behavior in production line pharmacies. Still, many pharmacies lean toward one approach or another when serving customers.

So, which approach is better? The answer depends on several factors:[9]

- *Basic business strategy.* If a pharmacy's business strategy is to provide low-cost, high-volume services, then a production line approach is preferred. If the business strategy is based on personalized, customized services, then an empowerment approach is better.
- *Nature of the transaction.* If most transactions between pharmacists and patients are single, discrete transactions, then a production line approach is better. If numerous transactions over a long time period lead to a pharmacist–patient therapeutic relationship, then an empowerment approach is preferred.
- *Needs of the patients.* Patients who have complex medical needs can benefit from services founded on an empowerment approach. If drug-related problems are routine and simple, a production line approach may be sufficient.
- *Type of employees and managers.* Each of these approaches works best with certain types of managers and employees. The production line approach works better for managers who prefer to monitor and control employees. Such managers may not feel comfortable sharing responsibility with employees. The production line approach also works when employees do not want to be empowered. Some pharmacy employees are more comfortable working in production line jobs that consist of routine tasks, easy-to-solve problems, and no-risk situations. The empowerment approach demands managers who are willing and able to help employees accept greater responsibility. This requires excellent leadership and coaching skills. In addition, the empowerment approach requires employees who want to take responsibility for their jobs and are bored and unchallenged by repetitive, routine tasks.

The answer to which approach is better comes down to a tradeoff between management control over the service process and employee involvement in services.[9] If management believes that greater control over the process will result in better customer value, then a production line approach may be preferable. On the other hand, if greater employee involvement in services is desired, then an empowerment approach should be used.

PLANNING FOR SERVICE PERFORMANCE

The quality of pharmacy services can be enhanced through better planning and design.[16] Two common strategies used in the design of services are presented here: service scripts and service blueprints.

Service Scripts

Businesses use service scripts to teach employees how to perform service duties and to standardize aspects of performance. A service script is a written list of actions describing service performance.[17,18] The following example is a service script for handling a penicillin-allergic patient who presents a prescription for a cephalosporin.

1. A penicillin-allergic patient presents a cephalosporin prescription.
2. The pharmacist questions the patient about details of the allergy to ascertain
   • Whether the patient actually has an allergy and
   • The severity of the allergic reaction.
3. The pharmacist calls the physician to discuss
   • The risks of dispensing the drug,
   • Possible alternatives for the patient, and
   • Directions for the patient.
4. The pharmacist initiates the agreed-upon action plan and documents the plan on the prescription.

The service script establishes the expected actions and responsibilities of the parties involved in performing the service. This example defines the problem (i.e., a penicillin-allergic patient presenting a prescription for a drug that may cause an allergic reaction), lists steps to be taken to solve the problem, and assigns responsibility for each step. There is little doubt about what is expected of the pharmacist.

The service script standardizes how employees handle problems. Standardization can reduce confusion for both the service provider and the customer. Imagine what would happen if a pharmacist did not document physician consultation about a prescription. A co-worker might call a physician about a problem that had already been solved. This would waste both the physician's and the pharmacist's time and cause the physician to wonder about the pharmacist's competence.

Service scripts should reflect the best known methods for handling service situations. Scripts should be developed by experienced service employees who can share their expertise. Input should also be solicited from employees who might be expected to follow the scripts. The scripts themselves should be comprehensive enough to help guide the actions of employees without constraining their ability to take care of customers.

Service scripts can be used in both production line and empowerment organizations. The difference lies in how they are used. In production line organizations, service scripts can be used as strict guidelines for employee behavior when dealing with customers. Here, scripts are followed without change or judgment. In empowerment organizations, scripts are used as a tool for training employees in unfamiliar tasks. They are used to suggest behavior, not as instructions to be followed exactly as written. As employees gain experience with the scripted task, they should be encouraged to move beyond it—to inject their own personality and experience into the service performance. This leads the employee to interpret and redefine the script, just as an actor does with the script of a play.

Many pharmacy schools use scripts in teaching their students. One example is the Indian Health Service guidelines for counseling patients. These guidelines require asking patients three questions:[19]

1. What did the doctor tell you the medicine is for?
2. How did the doctor tell you to take the medicine?
3. What did the doctor tell you to expect?

This simple script helps new pharmacists learn how to acquire basic information from patients that can be used in therapeutic problem solving. With experience, pharmacists can develop their own interpretation of the script, based on their own practice setting.

Service scripts be used for almost any situation, including clinical problems and basic work activities. New pharmacists might benefit from scripts dealing with the following: a dispensing error, a situation that requires a physician to change a prescribed therapy, a nonformulary prescription, a prior authorization, a nursing administration error, a patient complaint about the price of a prescription, a drug incompatibility, a physician prescribing error, a drug allergy or drug interaction, a service mistake (e.g., overcharge), negotiation with co-workers, a difficult counseling situation, a patient with renal or hepatic insufficiency, or a hostile customer.

Planning for Service Recovery

Service Failures

Many organizations have scripts for dealing with failures in service. All of us have experienced bad service. We may have had to wait too long for service or received merchandise we did not order. Bad service is a fact of life in business.

Providing bad service can hurt a firm's image. People are more likely to remember bad service than good service.[20,21] Bad service colors customer impressions of a firm, leads to negative comments about the experience, and drives customers to competitors.[22]

Failures can occur at numerous points in the service delivery process. Events within a service experience that determine the customer's overall evaluation of the service are called *critical incidents*. Critical incidents that are perceived as negative by the customer are called service failures. Service failures in pharmacy include incorrect charges for merchandise, unusually slow service, out-of-stock drugs, rude and uncooperative employees, and dispensing errors.

Customers respond to service failures in a number of ways. One way is to complain. Customers who complain are those who care enough to let an organization know that they are dissatisfied with some aspect of service. Complainers can actually be an organization's best friends, because they pinpoint problems in the service system that could lead to the loss of customers. Only a small fraction of customers complain, however.

Dissatisfied customers who do not complain show their displeasure with service failures in other ways. One way is to quit doing business with the company. These customers may make a conscious decision to never patronize a business again, or they may gradually move their business to competitors over time. In worst-case scenarios, they retaliate by trying to hurt the business in some way. They may go out of their way to complain to others about the poor service (e.g., setting up a Web site to share service "horror stories" about a company), take legal action, or even resort to vandalism against the business.

Service Recovery

The costs of poor service can be significant, and many organizations develop ways to address the problem of service failure. One important strategy is to design systems that minimize the number of service failures. However, it is impossible to prevent all bad experiences, so most businesses have plans to minimize the impact of service failure. Service recovery refers to all actions taken by personnel in a firm in response to a service failure. For example, if a customer notices that you have overcharged him for a drug by $10, the problem may seem easy to solve. You will just correct the charge and everything will be OK. Although your action may fix the problem, it won't necessarily win the customer back. The customer may assume that if you are sloppy with charges, you also may be sloppy in filling prescriptions. As a result, he probably will be wary of you and may withhold any further business.

When a service failure does occur, most service recovery programs use the following steps to help the customer feel good about doing business in the future:[13,14,23]

1. *Offer an apology.* When making an apology, first acknowledge that an error has been made and then acknowledge any inconvenience or anxiety it has caused. This lets the patient know that you recognize his or her situation and are concerned. Then take responsibility for remedying the situation. No matter who made the error or why it was made, you must convey concern for the customer and willingness to resolve the problem. Customers usually are not interested in reasons for the problem. What most people want to hear is, simply, "I'm truly sorry for the error."

2. *Offer a remedy.* Next, offer a remedy for the problem. It is important to follow up an apology with a solution that tells the customer you care about his or her well-being *and* future patronage. Listen to the customer's assessment of the problem, and find a solution that will address every concern the customer expresses. For example, if the customer seems to be concerned about future mischarges, explain how similar mistakes will be prevented.

3. *Fix the problem immediately.* Drop everything, and make solving this problem a priority. Doing so reinforces your dedication to resolving the problem and preserving the patient relationship. Acting assertively yet compassionately is crucial.

4. *Offer some form of compensation for the patient's inconvenience.* This step is not always necessary. For small failures, an apology may be enough. However, some compensation, such as forgoing a co-payment or filling the prescription at no charge, can let the customer know that (1) you consider the mistake unacceptable, (2) it won't happen again, and (3) you care about keeping his or her business. Companies that use compensation as part of their normal method of handling errors will either have to prevent errors from occurring or lose business through giveaways.

The surprising result of competent and sincere service recovery is that customers often feel better about the experience than if no service failure had occurred.[14] This is because failures give the service provider an opportunity to provide exceptional service. If the service provider performs well, the customer will recall the entire event in a positive light.

It is important to note that service recovery works only when service failures are rare. If a company has frequent failures in core services, customers will stop doing business with it, no matter what compensation is offered.

Service Blueprints[a]

The workflow in service organizations can have a tremendous impact on the quality and efficiency of services. Flowcharts called service blueprints are frequently used to map the steps of service delivery.

Service blueprints permit service providers to better see and understand service processes. A service blueprint depicts the process of service delivery and the roles of customers,

> *A service blueprint depicts the process of service delivery and the roles of customers, service providers, and supporting services.*

service providers, and supporting services. It breaks down the service into components and arranges them according to their purpose. Examples of service blueprints are shown in Figures 5-1 and 5-2.

Service blueprints are based on process design theory from industrial engineering, computer programming, decision theory, and operations management.[22,24] A key feature unique to service blueprinting is the inclusion of customers and their view of the process.[12] The premise of service blueprints is that if customers contribute to the service process, they should be recognized explicitly in its design and management. This means that the customer's "job" must be clearly defined.

The primary benefit of service blueprints is that they force a careful analysis of each step in the service process and communicate that information to people such as the frontline employees who help determine its success.

Components of a Service Blueprint

There are no concrete rules for designing service blueprints, so the process can be very flexible. However, service blueprints have some key components:[12] customer actions, "onstage" contact employee actions, "backstage" contact employee actions, and support processes, as shown in Figures 5-1 and 5-2.

Customer actions are performed by the customer, who can be any recipient of service (e.g., physician, nurse, patient), depending on the process. Customer actions in pharmacy include face-to-face consultation with pharmacists and telephone calls for prescription refills.

Customer actions are matched by onstage and backstage employee actions. Onstage employee actions are visible to the customer. The patient can see the pharmacist or technician taking the prescription and the pharmacist providing counseling. Anything done for the patient that

---

[a] This section was adapted from reference 16.

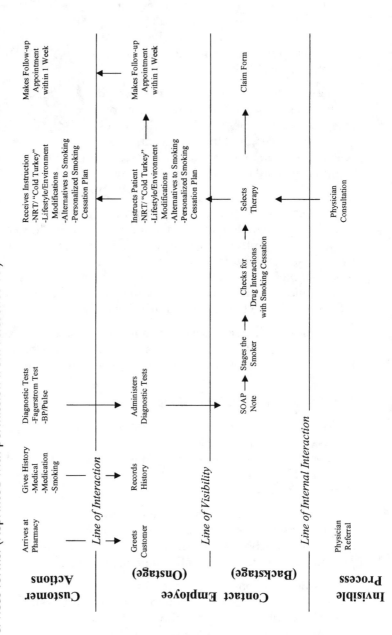

FIGURE 5-1 Service blueprint for a smoking cessation program. NRT = nicotine replacement therapy; SOAP = subjective and objective findings, assessment, and plan. "Claim Form" refers to the National Community Pharmacists Association pharmacist claim form and Centers for Medicare and Medicaid Services forms. (Reprinted with permission from reference 16.)

FIGURE 5-2 Service blueprint for dispensing services. DUR = drug-use review; RPh = pharmacist; Rx = prescription; tech = technician. (Reprinted with permission from reference 16.)

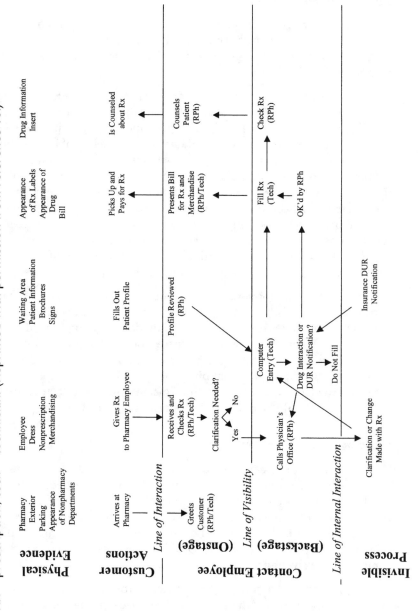

is not visible is a backstage employee action. Backstage actions include professional decisions made by pharmacists, such as checking the patient profile for drug allergies, interactions, and duplicate medications or consulting with the physician about therapy.

Support processes are those that support contact employees in the delivery of services. For pharmacists, these might include computer support services, billing, development of patient education inserts, and inventory control.

The service blueprint components are separated by three horizontal lines: the line of interaction, the line of visibility, and the line of internal interaction. The line of interaction is where customers and providers interact. Service encounters occur wherever a vertical line crosses the line of interaction. The line of visibility separates onstage contact employee actions and backstage employee actions. Actions below this line are invisible to the customer. This line is critical, because patients' image of a pharmacist is determined to a great extent by what they see the pharmacist do. If the primary patient view is of the pharmacist counting and pouring, then the image of pharmacists will be consistent with that view. The line of internal interaction separates frontline employees from supporting individuals. Any line that crosses this line indicates a process that supports the frontline employee.

An optional component of some service blueprints is physical evidence (see Figure 5-2). Customers often rely on tangible cues or physical evidence to evaluate services.[25] Physical evidence can include all features of the organization's physical structure and tangible communications: signs, parking, landscaping, lighting, cleanliness, decor, layout, and other visual cues. It is important that pharmacies control these aspects of a service experience, because they communicate a message to the customer. The message should be one that the pharmacy wants to send.

Building a Blueprint

Before a blueprint can be designed, a service process must be selected. An entire service process (e.g., dispensing) can be mapped, or the focus can be on a specific component of the process (e.g., patient counseling). An overview of the entire service process is called a *concept blueprint*.[26] Concept blueprints demonstrate how each job or department functions in relation to the process as a whole. *Detailed blueprints* can be used to clarify components identified in the concept blueprint.

Insight and understanding are gained through the development of a service blueprint.[12] Building a blueprint requires those involved to explicitly evaluate each step in the service process. This analysis encourages communication between designers, with several possible benefits. It can help clarify the service steps and identify obstacles that were not initially apparent. It can also help delineate the roles and responsibilities of each participant in the service process, even those who are not traditionally thought of as participants (e.g., customers, supporting services). Finally, it can foster a shared vision among all involved.

Since pharmacy blueprints encompass customers, pharmacists, technicians, managers, and supporting staff, all of these people should have input in blueprint development. Most critical, however, is understanding how customers view a service. A customer focus permits designers to highlight processes that accentuate customer value.

There are five steps to building a service blueprint:[12]

1. *Identify the process to be blueprinted.* Service blueprints should be designed with a specific purpose in mind. A concept blueprint might be used for understanding an overall process. To address specific problem areas of a service, a detailed blueprint might be more appropriate.
2. *Map the process from the customer's point of view.* Each action and choice of the customer is charted—not only those steps involved in purchasing a service but also those involved in consuming and evaluating it. This helps focus on the processes that affect customer perceptions.
3. *Map contact employee actions.* Mapping both onstage and backstage employee actions provides an opportunity for service employees and managers to communicate. Care must be taken to ensure that each term in the service blueprint has the same meaning for everyone, especially if there is opportunity for different interpretations. For example, it may be wise to define "patient counseling" in any blueprint. A line of interaction and a line of visibility should be drawn separating customer and employee actions and onstage and backstage employee actions, respectively.
4. *Map internal support activities.* The line of internal interaction should be drawn, and linkages between contact and support employees should be diagrammed.
5. *Add evidence of service at each customer action step.* The physical evidence of service can be mapped to illustrate what the customer sees and experiences during each contact with the pharmacy.

A service blueprint helps pharmacy managers identify potential problem areas in the service process. For example, a concept blueprint of a typical dispensing process for a new prescription in a community pharmacy is shown in Figure 5-2. If a community pharmacy manager finds that staff pharmacists are having difficulty counseling every patient who presents a new prescription, a review of this blueprint can help the manager figure out what the problem is. The manager can check each step in the

counseling process for potential obstacles. The manager may discover that the
pharmacist is not delegating tasks to the
technician and therefore is not leaving
adequate time for counseling. Or the
manager may find that pharmacists are
spending too much time clarifying new

> *Pharmacy services must be designed with customer value and satisfaction in mind.*

prescriptions or responding to unimportant computer drug-use review
notifications. The blueprint allows the pharmacist to see each step in the
process, probe for difficulties, and identify problem areas.

A blueprint also facilitates analysis of cost–benefit tradeoffs in designing
services. For example, the level of pharmacist–customer contact is critical.
A pharmacy that stresses efficiency in services may find it efficient to limit
patient–pharmacist interactions, because pharmacists can complete more
work when they are not interrupted by telephone calls and patient questions.
On the other hand, a customer-driven pharmacy may find that the greater
the contact, the greater is the opportunity to develop a patient relationship
and demonstrate the value of pharmacist services. The blueprint provides a
template for quantifying the value of patient contact, as measured by repeat
customers, patient satisfaction, and outcomes of drug therapy.

A blueprint also helps employees visualize the entire service process.
It enables each employee to better understand his or her role in the process, how that role affects others in the process, and exactly what is to be
achieved by everyone on the team. Including employees in the blueprinting process can increase their buy-in to operational changes or new service development by giving them the opportunity to provide feedback in
the planning stages instead of during implementation.

Pharmacy services must be designed with customer value and satisfaction in mind. Each design step should be assessed for its contribution
to the customer's perception of value, as well as its contribution to positive
patient outcomes. Steps that do not provide value should be reconsidered
or omitted.

SERVICE AUDITS

Service audits are another tool for improving the quality of services
within organizations. They are systematic, critical reviews of the way
organizations market services. The purpose of a service audit is to identify strengths and weaknesses of an organization's marketing efforts.[27]
Audits can be conducted by personnel within the organization or by critical, objective outsiders. Five important dimensions of services marketing
are included in service audits.

Marketing orientation refers to the degree to which marketing activities are important to the organization. The role of marketing research, management interaction with customers, the importance of marketing in managerial decisions, and similar issues are considered. Firms with a marketing orientation are in tune with the needs of customers.

New customer marketing refers to the degree to which attracting new customers is a priority for an organization. Efforts to attract customers and commitment to such efforts are examined.

Existing customer marketing refers to the degree to which keeping current customers is a priority. Formal efforts directed toward current customers and commitment to such efforts are considered, as well as actions taken to establish long-term relationships with customers.

Internal marketing refers to the degree to which the organization uses marketing concepts to attract, train, motivate, and retain high-quality employees. Employee recruitment activities, training, employee–management communication, and efforts to enhance employee satisfaction are assessed.

Service quality refers to the extent to which an organization is perceived by customers as providing excellent service that meets or exceeds expectations. Customer perceptions of reliability, responsiveness, and other dimensions of service quality are examined.

SUMMARY

Service design can make the difference between poor and excellent pharmacy services. The production line and empowerment approaches to the provision of services can both be useful frameworks. The choice of approach depends on the basic business strategy, the nature of the pharmacy transaction, the needs of patients, and the people employed by the pharmacy.

No matter which approach is chosen, pharmacists can benefit from techniques developed in other service industries. Service scripts can be developed to establish the expected actions and responsibilities of service employees. Service blueprints can be used to map the steps involved in service delivery. Service audits provide systematic, critical reviews of the role and performance of marketing within organizations.

References

1. Kenagy JW, Berwick DM, Shore MF. Service quality in health care. *JAMA.* 1999;281:661–5.
2. Chase RB, Hayes RH. Beefing up operations in service firms. *Sloan Manage Rev.* Fall 1991:15–26.

3. Bowen DE, Lawler EE. The empowerment of service workers: what, why, how and when. *Sloan Manage Rev.* Spring 1992:31–9.

4. Levitt T. Production line approach to service. *Harv Bus Rev.* September–October 1972:41–52.

5. Levitt T. Industrialization of service. *Harv Bus Rev.* September–October 1976:63–74.

6. Posey LM. Pushing the envelope: VA's mail-service operation. *J Am Pharm Assoc.* 1997;NS37:291–5.

7. Thompson CA. Mail-order services send out clinical services. *Am J Health Syst Pharm.* 1997;54:613,618,620,623.

8. Berry LL. On great service: a framework for action. *J Mark.* 1998;62:123–5.

9. Bowen DE, Lawler EE. Empowering service employees. *Sloan Manage Rev.* 1995;36:73–84.

10. Rafiq M, Ahmed PK. A customer-oriented framework for empowering service employees. *J Serv Mark.* 1998;12:379–96.

11. Schlesinger LA, Heskett JL. Breaking the cycle of failure in services. *Sloan Manage Rev.* Spring 1991:17–28.

12. Zeithaml VA, Bitner M. *Services Marketing.* New York: McGraw-Hill Co Inc; 1996.

13. Miller JL, Craighead CW, Karwan KR. Service recovery: a framework and empirical investigation. *J Oper Manage.* 2000;18:387–400.

14. Tax SS, Brown SW. Recovering and learning from service failure. *Sloan Manage Rev.* 1998;40:75–89.

15. Holdford DA. Evaluation of the Adequacy of Current Medicaid Reimbursement Rates as They Relate to Cognitive Services Provided by Pharmacists. Budget Bill item 322 #4b. 1998. (Virginia Department of Medical Assistance Services Study requested by Virginia State Legislature.)

16. Holdford DA, Kennedy DT. Service blueprint as a tool for designing innovative pharmaceutical services. *J Am Pharm Assoc.* 1999;39:545–52.

17. Shoemaker S. Scripts: precursor of consumer expectations. *Cornell Hotel Restaurant Adm Q.* February 1996:42–53.

18. Weiss WH. *Manager's Script Book.* Paramus, NJ: Prentice Hall; 1990.

19. Foster SL, Smith EB, Seybold MR. Advanced counseling techniques: integrating assessment and intervention. *Am Pharm.* 1995;NS35:40–8.

20. Mittal V, Ross WT, Baldasare PM. The asymmetric impact of negative and positive attribute-level performance on overall satisfaction and repurchase intentions. *J Mark.* 1998;62:33–47.

21. Mittal V, Lassar WM. Why do customers switch? The dynamics of satisfaction versus loyalty. *J Serv Mark.* 1998;12:177–94.

22. Zeithaml VA, Berry LL, Parasuraman A. The behavioral consequences of service quality. *J Mark.* 1996;60:31–46.

23. Maxham JG III. Service recovery's influence on consumer satisfaction, positive word-of-mouth, and purchase intentions. *J Bus Res.* 2001;54:11–24.

24. Shostack GL. Designing services that deliver. *Harv Bus Rev.* January–February 1984:133–9.

25. Bitner MJ. Servicescapes: the impact of physical surroundings on customers and employees. *J Mark.* 1992;56:57–61.

26. Kingman-Brundage J. The ABC's of service blueprinting. In: Bitner MJ, Crosby LA, eds. *Designing Winning Service Strategies.* Chicago: American Marketing Association; 1989:30–3.

27. Berry L, Conant JS, Parasuraman A. A framework for conducting a services marketing audit. *J Acad Mark Sci.* 1991;19:255–68.

Additional Readings

Bates DW. A 40-year-old woman who noticed a medication error. *JAMA.* 2001;285:3134–40.

Chase RB, Stewart DM. Make your service fail-safe. *Sloan Manage Rev.* 1994; 5(3):35–44.

Holdford DA. Service scripts—a tool for teaching pharmacy students how to handle common practice situations. *Am J Pharm Educ.* 2006;70(1):1–7.

John J. A dramaturgical view of the health care service encounter: cultural value-based impression management guidelines for medical professional behaviour. *Eur J Mark.* 1996;30:60–74.

Exercises and Questions

1. What approach to service design is most common in your work setting—the production line or empowerment approach? Explain your answer.
2. Could a production line approach to service design be consistent with the provision of pharmaceutical care? Why or why not?
3. How might service scripts be used in your pharmacy school to learn important skills? What skills should be learned through service scripts? When would a script not work?
4. How might pharmacists make some of their backstage performances more visible to patients and other customers?

Activities

1. Develop a script for what to say or do in one of the following service situations. Each person must choose a different situation. If it is useful in your practice setting, you may develop scripts for situations not listed here.
   - Dispensing error
   - Situation requiring a physician to change a prescribed therapy
   - Nonformulary prescription
   - Need for prior authorization
   - Nursing administration error
   - Patient complaint about the price of a prescription
   - Drug incompatibility
   - Physician prescribing error

- Drug allergy
- Drug interaction
- Service mistake (e.g., overcharge)
- Negotiation with co-workers
- Difficult counseling situation
- Patient with renal insufficiency
- Patient with hepatic insufficiency
- Hostile customer

2. Choose a service with which you are familiar and develop a service blueprint for it (e.g., dispensing a prescription). Identify activities that are hidden from the patient or other customer (e.g., nurse) and those that provide evidence for quality from the patient's viewpoint.

PART III

CONSUMER BEHAVIOR

CHAPTER **6**

CONSUMER BEHAVIOR

Objectives

After studying this chapter, the reader should be able to

❏ Describe the steps associated with consumer decision-making.
❏ Delineate how each step influences the choices consumers make.
❏ Discuss how risk, involvement, control, and expectations affect consumers' decision-making.
❏ Give a general description of the following models of health behavior: health belief model, theory of reasoned action, theory of planned behavior, and transtheoretical model.

All human actions have one or more of these seven causes: chance, nature, compulsions, habit, reason, passion, and desire.

Aristotle

Understanding the behavior of consumers is a fundamental requirement for marketing pharmacy products and pharmacist services. Good marketers realize how and why consumers make decisions about the purchase and use of drugs. Knowledge about consumer behavior is essential in setting prices, merchandising, advertising, designing services, and other marketing activities.

Decision-making in health care differs in several ways from consumer decisions about purchasing nonhealth products and services. The health care consumer (i.e., the patient) often does not choose the treatment to be consumed (e.g., the drug); that decision is left to the physician or other health care professional. Furthermore, patients usually pay directly only a fraction of the cost of health care. Most costs are paid by third-party payers such as insurance companies, employers, and the government. These third-party payers exert significant influence on consumer decisions.

Detailed discussion of the many decision makers in health care is beyond the scope of this book. This chapter focuses on decision-making by patients. Understanding patient decision-making is important for pharmacists because of the large number of consumer-generated pharmacy transactions (e.g., nonprescription and herbal products, general merchandise) and the expanding role of consumers in health care choices.

CONSUMER DECISIONS

Consumers make decisions to fulfill their unmet needs and wants. A patient goes to a pharmacy to satisfy some desire (e.g., treat a cold). The patient's decision about how to fulfill that desire is influenced by a variety of personal, social, and economic factors, such as perceptions of risk and recommendations from friends. The following paragraphs describe three frameworks for understanding consumer behavior.[1]

Economic man. Much of what marketers know about consumer behavior originates from economics. Economic understanding of consumer behavior is based in part on the assumptions that (1) people are rational in their behavior, (2) they attempt to maximize personal satisfaction through exchange, (3) they possess complete information on available alternatives, and (4) they use that information to make a choice. The model of economic man is useful in identifying behaviors relating to price, consumer income, quality, and consumer tastes. From economics, we know that demand for a drug is positively associated with low prices for the drug, high prices for drug substitutes, high consumer income, consumer tastes, and the quality of the drug and accompanying service.

However, economics makes many assumptions about consumers that are not borne out in real life. Often, consumers make choices irrationally (i.e., they act in ways that seem contrary to their best interests) and lack or ignore information that could be used in making choices. Furthermore, the classic economic man framework does not consider many cultural, social, and psychological influences on demand.

Social influences. Much of consumer behavior is influenced by our interactions with others. From birth, humans are influenced by subtle pressures that form our desires and actions. These pressures can emanate from social norms established by peer groups, reference groups, family, and social class. Much of our understanding of drug use is founded on social theories.

Personal influences. Each person is driven by a variety of desires and pressures that influence behavior. Complex psychological processes occur that are difficult for others to see but crucial to how we act. Consumer behavior is influenced by our personality, values, beliefs, and attitudes. As might be expected, much of what we know about personal influences comes from the field of psychology.

Marketers draw from these frameworks and many others to understand consumer behavior. Economics and social sciences provide the foundation of most marketing theory and practices. As a result, many processes in pharmaceutical marketing originate from other disciplines. For example, the marketing of interventions to increase patient adherence to drug regimens is largely based on our understanding of economic, social, and psychological behavior.

A variety of factors contribute to nonadherence to therapeutic regimens, frustrating health care providers' efforts to influence drug-taking behavior.[2] Economics has an obvious effect when patients have to pay all or a portion of the costs of the medications they consume. Social and demographic variables (age, sex, marital status, size of household, social class, attitudes of peers and family members) affect compliance in ways that may be hard to predict. Psychological and cognitive influences include the patient's knowledge, mental capability, beliefs about medicine, self-efficacy, and previous experiences. Noncompliance is a complex issue that requires sophisticated interventions by providers, who must integrate their knowledge of disease, therapies, and patient behaviors.

CONSUMER PURCHASE SITUATIONS

Consumer decisions fall into two categories: new and repeat decisions (Figure 6-1). The first visit to a pharmacy or the choice of a new cough and cold preparation would be a new decision. A visit to a pharmacy to refill a prescription or buy more nonprescription pain medication would be a repeat decision.

New decisions range from the complex to the simple. Complex decisions tend to involve extended problem solving and substantial consideration and effort by the consumer. Major health care decisions, such as a decision to undergo surgery, typically require extended problem solving. Limited problem solving is used for simple problems that can be handled without much mental effort. Impulse purchases (i.e., unplanned, spur-of-the-moment reactions to a presented product) are the least complex form of problem solving.

Repeat decisions also range from the complex to the simple, and they account for many consumer and health care decisions. Typically, repeat decisions require less contemplation than new decisions and can be handled with limited problem solving. Consumers use experience gained

FIGURE 6-1   Types of consumer decisions.

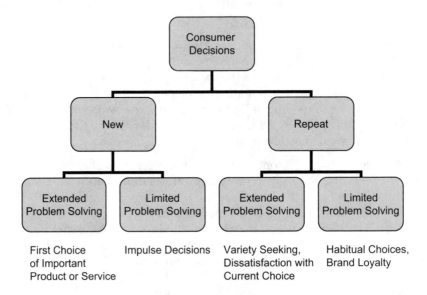

from previous decisions to simplify the purchase process. For example, patients often remain loyal to nonprescription cough and cold medications because they remember that previous use brought them relief. Rather than carefully weigh each alternative, the consumer simply chooses the brand that worked the last time.

Consumers' use of extended or limited problem solving depends on a variety of factors. Extended problem solving occurs more often with new, high-risk, and complex problems. It is more likely to be used by someone who is engaged in a first-time search for a drug to treat a severe, multisymptom cold than by someone in search of a frequently purchased headache medication. Extended problem solving is also more likely when the consumer has time for and interest in the decision. Busy consumers often do not have the luxury of time for detailed analysis of the options.

The degree to which patients engage in problem solving has important implications for pharmacists.[3] Patients who engage in extended problem solving want information to guide their decisions and are more likely to pay attention to longer, more thoughtful messages. Patients who engage in limited problem solving restrict their attention to short, repetitive messages with low information content.

FIGURE 6-2 Stages of consumer decision-making. (Compiled from reference 4.)

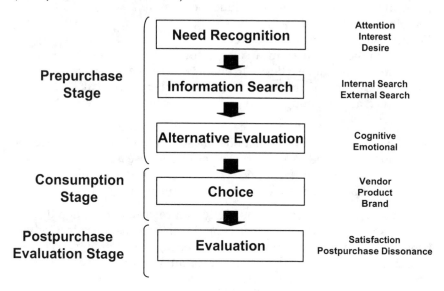

THE CONSUMER DECISION PROCESS

Numerous decision-making models have been proposed by marketers over the years. One widely accepted model, shown in Figure 6-2, has three major stages.[4] Prepurchase is the stage in which consumers recognize a need and identify choices to meet that need; it consists of need recognition, information search, and alternative evaluation. Consumption is the actual selection and purchase of a product. Postpurchase describes the evaluation phase of consumer decision-making.

This model can be used to describe decisions ranging from the simple (e.g., habitual and impulse buying) to the complex (e.g., deciding between surgery and drug therapy). Consumers may not consciously go through each step in the model. For instance, people who make impulse purchases frequently forgo the prepurchase and postpurchase stages.

Prepurchase

Need Recognition

Consumer decision-making begins with the recognition of a need. This occurs when some stimulus arouses a desire (e.g., a headache arouses a desire to get rid of the pain). Desire-arous-ing stimuli can be commercial, social, or physical.[4] Commercial stimuli include those commonly associated with the market-ing mix, such as a television advertisement or a recommendation from a salesperson.

> *Consumer decision-making begins with the recognition of a need.*

Social stimuli might be a desire to emulate one's peers or word-of-mouth recommendations of friends or family members. Physical stimuli are things such as pain, hunger, and thirst.

Marketers attempt to influence consumer need recognition in numer-ous ways. They develop promotional messages to directly stimulate the recognition of a need. An advertisement might pose a provocative ques-tion ("Are you getting the service you deserve?") or announce new ser-vices ("Bone mineral density testing now available").

Marketers also attempt to indirectly induce need recognition by sim-ulating social situations in advertising. Direct-to-consumer drug adver-tisements often portray attractive people engaged in activities related to drug consumption. An advertisement for an arthritis medication might show an older person playing tennis—the message being that the drug can help you be more active, like this person. A pharmacy advertisement might portray a patient using a computer to access Internet pharmacy ser-vices—the message being that it is easy and convenient.

Another way to indirectly induce need recognition is to use sounds, smells, and images to activate physical reactions that lead to consumer purchases. Anyone who has smelled freshly baked bread in a bakery or brewed coffee in a café recognizes the desire that can be stimulated by smells. Music is often piped into stores to affect moods and make con-sumers more likely to buy. The marketing term *servicescapes* describes the role of facility design features such as lighting, temperature, sound, and signs in influencing consumer behavior.[5]

Despite the best efforts of marketers, however, most stimuli are inef-fective in causing need recognition. That is because most are not even noticed. Humans ignore most stimuli, because we are constantly bom-barded by commercial messages, social demands, and physical aches and pains. Ignoring them is the only way to survive in this message-laden world. Because people are selective in their attention to stimuli, marketers continually look for innovative ways to break through all of the environ-mental noise.

To complicate matters for marketers, stimuli that arouse attention do not always arouse sufficient desire to cause action. A smoker may notice and be interested in an advertisement for a smoking cessation program, but the ad may not be sufficient to get the smoker to take action (i.e., enroll in the program). Smokers are continually exposed to commercial, social, and physical messages telling them to quit, but they fail to do so for many reasons, including the perception that the effort it would take to quit is too great.

Information Search

Once a need is recognized, a consumer goes through a search for information about actions that might meet the perceived need or want. This can be a simple search of one's memory (called an *internal search*), in which previous experiences or promotional messages are recalled. For instance, a patient who wants information about a nonprescription medication might search her memory for experience with particular brands or information relayed through a television advertisement.

In many cases, the internal memory search is followed by an *external search* for information. In the nonprescription medication example, a patient might consult a friend, an issue of *Consumer Reports* magazine, the Internet, or a pharmacist. The level of consumer search depends on several factors:[4]

Whether the decision is a new or repeat one. People who are unfamiliar with the available choices of products or services are more likely to engage in an external search. These people may be more attentive to promotional messages, ask others for recommendations, or engage in research in consumer publications or on the Internet.

Whether products and services are perceived to be different. There is little need for a search when a choice will result in essentially the same outcome. A patient who perceives all pharmacies and pharmacists to be the same will see little reason to engage in an extensive search for a pharmacy. The search may involve simply recalling where the nearest pharmacy is located.

Individual situations and characteristics. Individuals who lack the time or ability to evaluate information are less likely to engage in a search. Busy people are less likely to spend time choosing nonprescription medications in a community pharmacy. Personal knowledge also influences the level of the search. Individuals with less knowledge of health care are more likely to rely on the opinions of others than to engage in their own search for information.

Several strategies can be used to influence the information search. One is to establish your product or service firmly in the minds of consumers through advertising and other promotional communication (see

Chapter 11). When this has been accomplished, your product or service will be considered in the consumer's internal memory search. Another strategy is to guide consumers through the external search process with questions and statements such as the following:

- Did your pharmacist check for interactions?
- Not all medicines are alike. Have you ever considered drug *y*?
- If you have never used drug *x*, here is what you need to know.
- Are you completely happy with drug *x*? If not, try drug *y*.
- Do you ever worry that you are paying too much for drug *x*?

Evaluation of Alternatives

Once sufficient information has been collected, the consumer can evaluate alternatives. The evaluation can be cognitive (thoughtful), or it can be noncognitive (emotional). Cognitive evaluation of alternatives involves contemplation and thought. Most consumer behavior models assume a cognitive process. Noncognitive evaluation is less thoughtful, involving intuition or gut feelings.

Noncognitive decisions about care have a greater impact than health professionals may realize. Patients typically choose drugs and health care providers on the basis of feelings, not thoughts. If we have a headache, we don't select a remedy by objective cost–benefit analysis; we simply choose a drug to stop the pain so we can continue what we were doing before the headache began. Our choice of a pharmacist is likely to be determined less by her technical capability than by our feelings when she reassures us about our condition, conveys that she cares about us as people, and helps us feel in control of our health. Even an objective attribute such as low cost may appeal to us more because we feel we are getting a good deal than because of the actual impact on our budget. Many times, our preferences concerning the appearance and features of products and services are based on feelings rather than thoughtful analysis of the pros and cons.

In any evaluation of alternatives, the first step is to identify the important criteria or attributes, such as price and quality of services. This can be difficult for consumers with little knowledge of or experience with the available alternatives. Free trials of products or services provide consumers with some experience. As an added benefit, free trials may encourage consumers to share their experiences with others.

Decisions between alternatives often are based on more than one attribute; this is called multiattribute decision-making. Table 6-1 illustrates a consumer's use of the attributes price, location, and pharmacist

TABLE 6-1 Consumer Assessment of Community Pharmacies

Attribute	Pharmacy A	Pharmacy B	Pharmacy C
Price	Highest in town but still competitive	Competitive	Lowest in town
Location	Near home	Near home and work	Across town
Pharmacist relationship	Excellent and long lasting	No relationship	No relationship

relationship to choose a pharmacy. This consumer has chosen to consider only three attributes, possibly because of time limitations or unwillingness to invest more effort in the decision.

After choosing which attributes to consider, the consumer weighs the relative importance of each and examines how the attributes differ among alternatives (i.e., the competing pharmacies). Some attributes are more important or salient in decision-making than others. Price may be more salient to some consumers, while location or pharmacist relationship may be more salient to others. Clear differences between salient attributes can influence the selection of one alternative over another.

On the other hand, important attributes may have little effect on the final choice. For instance, low drug prices might be expected to be salient in the selection of a pharmacy, but this attribute may be irrelevant to the final choice if the consumer perceives no price difference between competitors. In fact, the widespread use of prescription drug insurance has lessened the role of drug prices as a driver of pharmacy choice.[6]

The attributes that are perceived to differ enough between the alternatives to influence the final choice are called *determinant attributes*. The alternatives being considered may differ little in regard to highly salient attributes. Competing pharmacies may be similar in regard to price and convenience. In this case, the choice of a pharmacy can depend on seemingly less important attributes (e.g., neatness, lighting). Good pharmacists pay attention to even minor details when it comes to service, because those details can make the final difference in patient patronage and loyalty.

In Table 6-1, Pharmacy A is the most expensive, but it is near home and the patient has a good relationship with the pharmacist. Pharmacy B has competitive prices and is near work and home, but the patient has no relationship with the pharmacist. Pharmacy C has the lowest prices, but it is across town and again there is no pharmacist relationship. Pharmacy patronage will depend on individual preference.

The reasons for patients' choice of a pharmacy have been studied extensively over the years.[6-8] The research has identified many attributes as salient: convenient location, the pharmacist, patient out-of-pocket cost, convenient hours, friendliness of employees, personalized attention, and specialized services. Attributes that are beyond the control of most pharmacists, such as convenience (i.e., location, operating hours) and out-of-pocket costs to patients, may be determinant. However, pharmacists have the power to influence attributes such as friendliness, personalized attention, professional services, and reliability of care. The extent to which these attributes can determine pharmacy patronage depends on patients, situational factors, and the attributes of competing pharmacies.

Consumption Stage

Choice

The prepurchase stage, as described above, prepares consumers for the next stage: making a choice. In truth, consumer choice may consist of several choices. Choosing a nonprescription drug involves choosing a vendor (e.g., drugstore, grocery, mass merchandiser), a channel of distribution (e.g., drive-through, mail order, or Internet pharmacy), and a brand (e.g., generic, store brand, manufacturer brand).

The consumption stage extends beyond product selection and purchase. It also includes the use and disposal of the product. The consumption process for a prescription medication encompasses all consumer actions related to the purchase, use, and disposal of the drug. These include selecting a pharmacy, filling and paying for the prescription, taking the medication, and throwing away any medication that has not been consumed.

Decision Rules

Once consumers have determined which criteria to use in making a decision, they make overall judgments based on the criteria and compare them across alternatives. Typically, these judgments follow personal decision rules that the consumer develops through experience.

One consumer decision rule is to apply cutoffs[4]—strict limits for deciding which choices are acceptable and unacceptable. Setting a defined price range (e.g., no more than $10) is a common cutoff rule used by consumers. Prices that fall outside the established range are judged unacceptable.

The application of absolute cutoff rules to decisions is called *noncompensatory decision-making*. Noncompensatory means that deficiencies in some attributes cannot be compensated for by strengths in others. Hence, a product or service with an unacceptable price will not be considered, no matter how favorable the other attributes may be.

Cutoffs can be applied to pharmacy selection. Limits might be established for the distance to a pharmacy, the behavior of pharmacy personnel, and the range of products offered. The use of cutoffs can simplify the decision-making process, but often consumers are left with multiple alternatives that have passed the cutoff rule. Additional decision rules must be used to choose among the remaining alternatives.

Another decision rule used by consumers is to sum the value of the attributes into an overall value for each option. The option with the greatest overall value (i.e., utility) is chosen. Marketers call choices based on overall utility *compensatory decisions*.[4] In compensatory decision-making, the weaknesses of one attribute can be overcome by the strength of another. Thus, consumers may be willing to accept high prices for pharmaceutical services if the quality of those services is perceived to result in significant value.

Postpurchase Evaluation

Once consumption is completed, consumers evaluate the decision-making process. They evaluate the degree to which their needs and wants have been met, as well as their overall satisfaction with the experience. What was received is compared with what was expected.

During this stage, consumers often have doubts about their choices. They experience *cognitive dissonance*, particularly when a bad choice could have serious consequences, such as placing personal or financial health at significant risk. Cognitive dissonance is common after people buy an expensive car or a house. They may worry about whether they can afford the purchase and what would happen if something went wrong with what they have bought.

Cognitive dissonance can occur after making health care decisions. Patients may worry about the expense or potential adverse effects associated with a choice. Pharmacists can minimize patients' cognitive dissonance in several ways. One is to make telephone calls to patients a day or two after filling a prescription. This gives the patient an opportunity to communicate concerns to the pharmacist and seek reassurance. Another is to include a notice in the prescription package that encourages the patient to call the pharmacy with questions or visit a Web site for answers to commonly asked questions. Some pharmacies even make money-back guarantees to patients.

VARIABLES AFFECTING CONSUMER DECISION-MAKING

> *Decisions are influenced by the consumer's tolerance for risk.*

Perception of Risk

Decisions are influenced by the consumer's tolerance for risk. A risk taker is likely to act differently than a risk avoider. Five types of perceived risk have been defined.[9]

1. Financial risk refers to financial losses that might occur as a result of a bad purchase, such as overpaying for a nonprescription drug or finding out that a prescription drug is not covered by insurance.
2. Performance risk is the possibility that a purchase will not achieve the intended outcome, such as when an allergy drug does not relieve allergic symptoms.
3. Physical risk is the potential for injury resulting from consumption. For drugs, this might refer to adverse effects or drug interactions.
4. Social risk refers to loss of personal social status associated with a purchase. Some drugs, such as those used to treat urinary incontinence or AIDS, can carry a stigma.
5. Psychological risk refers to the impact of a purchase on a person's self-esteem. Some drugs have potentially embarrassing adverse effects, such as impotence or flatulence, that can negatively affect self-esteem.

Decisions about health care, including medication use, are perceived to be riskier than the average consumer purchase decision. The perception of risk has two dimensions: severity and chance.[10] Severity refers to the significance of possible consequences of a decision. With decisions about medications, negative consequences can range in severity from none to pain, suffering, and even death. The greater the severity of a potential outcome, the greater is the risk associated with the decision. Chance refers to the probability of a certain outcome occurring. For drugs, uncertainty about effectiveness, adverse effects, and drug interactions increases the perception of risk.

Evaluating the risk involved in using pharmacy products and pharmacist services is difficult for most consumers. They lack both the expertise to decide which medications will help their conditions and information on how to use them appropriately. Even after taking a medication, consumers may not know whether it is working unless they receive feedback from the health care provider. Patients need providers to tell them if their cholesterol levels or liver enzymes are too high.

Involvement

Involvement is defined as the consumer's perception of the importance of a person, object, or situation.[4] It describes an internal state of arousal, preparedness, and attention. Involvement is an indicator of motivation because it signals personal relevance. Sick people pay more attention to health messages than healthy

> *Decisions about health care, including medication use, are perceived to be riskier than the average consumer purchase decision.*

people do, because the messages are more relevant to their personal situation. The degree of consumer involvement can vary from moment to moment, depending on a person's changing situation.

Involvement is an important concept for pharmacists, because consumers who are interested in their health and health care behave differently than those who are not. Involvement is positively related to extended problem solving. Interested consumers are more alert to health information, committed to their therapeutic plan, and likely to work with professionals to achieve good therapeutic outcomes. In addition, involvement is important because it influences consumer decision-making.

The information search, information processing, and susceptibility to persuasion are affected by the consumer's involvement.[4] Involved consumers spend more time and effort searching for information that relates to purchase and consumption. They are more thoughtful in their actions, understand information better, and have greater ability to recall details later. Also, involved people are more likely to listen to persuasive arguments.

Involvement is necessary for thoughtful behavior, which is needed when dealing with important, complex decisions such as those about health care. Participation in health care decision-making requires consumers to fully understand their choices and the consequences. This means consumers should be attentive to information and thoughtful in their choices. Consumers who are not thoughtful are more likely to make decisions on the basis of emotions, habit, or random choice. Involvement with pharmaceuticals and pharmacy services is influenced by several factors:[4]

- *Personal relevance of the object to the consumer.* Although pharmacists may perceive their services as critically important, patients may not consider these services crucial. The relevance of anything is determined by the perspective of the individual.

- *The product or service being considered.* Some things are inherently more important to people than others. Health care is considered a high-involvement activity in comparison with the purchase of a commodity such as laundry detergent. Involvement with health care is related to the perceived risk associated with its purchase and consumption and the potential benefit it can provide to meet personal needs. The more aware people are of the potential benefit or risk associated with specific health care decisions, the greater will be their attention and involvement.
- *The situation.* Many healthy people ignore health care issues—until they get sick. Then they become actively involved in finding a way to treat their illness. Their involvement is situation dependent. When the illness is resolved, the need for involvement changes, and the person may fall back to his or her previous low level of involvement.

Involvement in Pharmacy Services

In general, consumers are involved in decisions relating to pharmacist services and pharmacy products. Arneson et al.[11] found that significant numbers of pharmacy patients are highly concerned about their health care needs, the medications they purchase, and the professional services they receive. Lipowski[12] found that people are involved with prescription products more than with other goods. Holdford and Watrous[3] showed that consumers realize the importance of pharmacy services and are only slightly less involved with pharmacist services than with physician services.

Lipowski states that expertise and opportunity are important for patient involvement in decisions about drugs and pharmaceutical services. She suggests that consumers must have sufficient expertise and opportunity to engage in the thoughtful decisions involved in the provision of pharmaceutical care. Thus, patients who gain sufficient knowledge of and familiarity with their drugs (i.e., expertise) and the ability to comprehend and use this information (i.e., opportunity) will be more involved in their health care decisions.

Customizing Services to Patient Involvement

Pharmacists who understand their patients' level of involvement can use that knowledge to tailor educational and counseling information and stimulate greater involvement.[3] Standardized surveys are available for measuring involvement, but they are rarely necessary. Most pharmacists can assess a patient's involvement level by observing body language, eye contact, and responses to questions about treatments.

Patients who are highly involved can receive more complex messages and greater amounts of information. These patients will be receptive and pay attention. Persuasive messages are more effective with involved patients, because the patients are more willing to follow the logic and information associated with persuasive arguments.

For low-involvement patients, relatively simple, short, repetitive messages are better. A smaller amount of information should be provided in plain language. Repetition of crucial messages helps low-involvement patients retain information long enough for it to influence their behavior.

Enhancing Patient Involvement

Pharmacists can enhance their patients' involvement and help make them more receptive to the complex health messages that are commonly part of the practice of pharmaceutical care. Greater involvement can be stimulated in the following ways:[3]

- Expertise can be increased by educating patients about their diseases and medication therapy. Pharmacists can convey to patients the role of pharmacy services in achieving positive health outcomes.
- Opportunity to process information can be enhanced by reducing the number of distractions and providing a quiet counseling area for conversations with patients. Opportunity can also be increased by scheduling patient counseling sessions at hours convenient for both the pharmacist and the patient.
- When patients have limited expertise and opportunity, pharmacists should adjust counseling strategies to the patient's level. Pharmacists should provide only as much information as the patient can adequately process and should simplify the message for patients with less education or reduced cognitive ability.

Pharmacists need to understand consumer involvement, because it affects the way information is processed. For medication counseling to be effective, the patient must receive and understand the message being conveyed by the pharmacist. Insufficient mental involvement of the patient in the counseling transaction can lead to misunderstanding and ultimate therapeutic failure.

Perception of Control

Control refers to consumers' perceptions that they can influence their personal situations and environment. Control is a fundamental desire of

humans, and low levels of control are associated with high levels of stress. In pharmacists, lack of control is associated with job
burnout.[13]

It is important for consumers to feel that they control the pharmacy service experience.

It is important for consumers to feel that
they control the pharmacy service experience. Consumers who sense that they lack
control are more likely to become dissatisfied and act to regain control.
Consumers who see a long checkout line in a pharmacy may exert control
by attempting to find another checkout line, continue shopping until the
line becomes shorter, or leave the pharmacy without making a purchase.

Marketers use several strategies to increase a consumer's feeling of
control. One is to provide detailed feedback about the consumer's progress in the service sequence. This helps the consumer know what will
happen next and how long it will take to complete the process. Feedback
about the service process helps consumers reset overoptimistic expectations and enables them to make an informed choice about whether to wait.
Then, a 30-minute wait to fill a prescription becomes a conscious choice
rather than something that is inflicted upon them.

Another strategy is to increase choice. Consumers who can select
among various options feel more in control. However, too many options
can make consumers feel overwhelmed and frustrated. Two or three alternatives are usually sufficient.

Finally, marketers often try to make service experiences as consistent
and predictable as possible. At most chain pharmacies or mass merchandisers, consumers find little variation among stores. That is because consumers like to know that the CVS or Walgreens in a distant town will be
similar to the one in their neighborhood. The ability to find merchandise
and services at any store gives consumers the perception of control over
their purchase and the service experience.

HEALTH BEHAVIOR MODELS

In addition to the three-stage model of consumer behavior discussed
in the preceding sections, other models can help pharmacists understand
health behaviors.

Health Belief Model

The health belief model is one of the best known and most widely
studied models of health behavior. It has been applied to adherence to
therapy, smoking behavior, and participation in preventive health care.[14]

It has also been used to develop a fundamental understanding of drug-use behaviors.[15,16] The health belief model states that the consumer's likelihood of taking action to prevent or treat a health condition is determined by his or her perception of susceptibility to that condition, the severity of the condition, the benefits of taking action, the costs of taking action, and the barriers to taking action.[17]

Health care interventions should attempt to address each of these five factors in order to influence consumer behavior. The consumer should be targeted with some cue to action (e.g., an educational pamphlet or television advertisement) that heightens his or her perception of susceptibility to the condition, the severity of the condition, and the benefits of taking action. The cue should also attempt to modify perceptions about the costs of and barriers to taking action.

Theories of Reasoned Action and Planned Behavior

The theory of reasoned action and the theory of planned behavior have similar origins. The theory of reasoned action states that intentions to act (e.g., "How likely are you to quit smoking?") are predictive of actual consumer behavior.[18] Intentions to act, in turn, are determined by a person's positive or negative attitude toward performing that act ("How desirable is smoking for you?") and the person's assessment of social pressures toward action ("How do your family members feel about your smoking behavior?"). Attitudes are determined by beliefs about the consequences of an action ("I will gain weight if I stop smoking") and the perceived importance of those consequences ("Gaining weight will make me look fat").

Social pressures (i.e., subjective norms) are determined by the expectations of others ("My spouse really wants me to quit") weighted by the perceived importance of the opinions of others. Therefore, changing behavior starts with influencing beliefs, attitudes, and intentions about a behavior through education and persuasive messages.

The theory of planned behavior adds to the theory of reasoned action by addressing the issue of control over behavior.[19] Behavioral control associated with personal resources, capabilities, opportunity, and desire modifies the impact of social pressures and attitude on intentions to act.

Although the link between intentions and behavior is not always strong, there is evidence in the pharmacy literature to support the value of the theory of reasoned action in explaining influences on physician uses of drug information[20] and patient compliance with medication regimens.[21] The theory of planned behavior has been applied to the study of herbal medicine use by older patients. [22]

Transtheoretical Model

The transtheoretical model of behavior change has been used to predict pharmacists' readiness to provide pharmaceutical care[23] and patients' readiness to quit smoking.[24] According to this model, people progress through five stages of change; the success of behavior-change strategies depends on what stage the person is in.[25]

In stage 1, precontemplation, the consumer has no intention of changing in the foreseeable future. In fact, the consumer is resistant to interventions designed to cause immediate change. The consumer may be unaware of or in denial about a need for change.

In stage 2, contemplation, the consumer has some intention to change in the foreseeable future but is still unwilling to take immediate action. The consumer is aware of a problem but has not yet made the commitment to action.

In stage 3, preparation, the consumer has begun to take small steps toward making a change in the very near future. These might consist of searching for information about therapeutic choices or making an appointment with a health care professional.

In stage 4, action, the consumer is taking active steps to make a change.

In stage 5, maintenance, the change has been made. The consumer now attempts to consolidate the success and avoid relapse into old behaviors.

On average, 40% to 60% of people in the process of change are in stage 1 or 2 (not ready to change any time in the near future). Nevertheless, efforts are often made to change their behavior, which may result in resistance to the intervention or temporary change and subsequent relapse. For example, smokers who are not ready to quit are more likely to make half-hearted efforts that result in failure.

Successful application of the transtheoretical model requires identifying the stage of change for each consumer. At stage 1 or 2, interventions should simply attempt to move the consumer to a higher stage of readiness. This can be done by increasing the perceived benefits of change and enhancing confidence that a change can successfully be made (e.g., by showing the consumer how to take baby steps that will result in small successes). For consumers in stages 3 and 4, efforts should be made to facilitate and reinforce change. This means giving people what they need in order to change, such as information, training, and support. For smoking cessation, this might consist of regularly scheduled counseling sessions with the quitter for education, coaching, and problem solving. In stage 5, interventions are used to manage the consumer's temptation to slide back into previous undesirable behavior.

SUMMARY

Understanding the behavior of consumers is an essential part of marketing pharmacy products and pharmacist services. Pharmacists can benefit from understanding some basic principles of consumer behavior. They can use this knowledge to influence patient medication compliance, change smoking behavior, advertise services, design services, and influence physician prescribing.

References

1. Bradley F. *Marketing Management: Providing, Communicating and Delivering Value.* Upper Saddle River, NJ: Prentice Hall; 1995.
2. Vermeire E, Hernshaw H, Van Royen P, et al. Patient adherence to treatment: three decades of research. A comprehensive review. *J Clin Pharm Ther.* 2001;26:331–42.
3. Holdford DA, Watrous ML. Relative importance consumers place on pharmaceutical services. *J Pharm Mark Manage.* 1997;11(4):55–68.
4. Engel JF, Blackwell RD, Miniard PW. *Consumer Behavior.* Fort Worth, Tex: Dryden Press; 1993.
5. Bitner MJ. Servicescapes: the impact of physical surroundings on customers and employees. *J Mark.* 1992;56:57–61.
6. Xu KT. Choice of and overall satisfaction with pharmacies among a community-dwelling elderly population. *Med Care.* 2002;40:1283–93.
7. Gagnon JP. Factors affecting pharmacy patronage motives—a literature review. *J Am Pharm Assoc.* 1977;NS17:556–9,566.
8. Duska F, Grauer DW, Law AV. An evaluation of patient attitudes toward pharmacy selection: a determinant attribute approach. *J Pharm Mark Manage.* 2005;17(1):35–50.
9. Kare A, Kucukarslan S, Birdwell S. Consumer perceived risk associated with prescription drugs. *Drug Inf J.* 1996;30:465–72.
10. Ganther J, Kreling DH. Consumer perceptions of risk and required cost savings for generic prescription drugs. *J Am Pharm Assoc.* 2000;40:378–83.
11. Arneson DL, Jacobs EW, Scott DM, et al. Patronage motives of community pharmacy patrons. *J Pharm Mark Manage.* 1989;4:3–22.
12. Lipowski E. How consumers choose a pharmacy. *J Am Pharm Assoc.* 1993; 33:S7–S14.
13. Gupchup GV, Singhal PK, Dole EF, et al. Burnout in a sample of HMO pharmacists using the Maslach burnout inventory. *J Manag Care Pharm.* 1998;4:495–503.
14. Mullen PD, Hersey JC, Iverson DC. Health behavior models compared. *Soc Sci Med.* 1987;24:973–81.
15. Cohen NL, Parikh SV, Kennedy SH. Medication compliance in mood disorders: relevance of the health belief model and other determinants. *Prim Care Psychiatry.* 2000;6:101–10.
16. Fincham JE, Wertheimer AI. Correlates and predictors of self-medication attitudes of initial drug therapy defaulters. *J Soc Admin Sci.* 1985;3:10–7.

17. Becker MH, Maiman LA. Sociobehavioral determinants of compliance with health and medical care recommendations. *Med Care.* January 1975;13: 10–24.
18. Ajzen I, Fishbein M. *Understanding Attitudes and Predicting Social Behavior.* Englewood Cliffs, NJ: Prentice Hall; 1980.
19. Ajzen I. The theory of planned behavior. *Organ Behav Hum Decis Process.* 1991;50:179–211.
20. Gaither CA, Bagozzi RP, Ascione FJ, et al. Reasoned action approach to physicians' utilization of drug information sources. *Pharm Res.* 1996;13: 1291–8.
21. Ried LD, Christensen D. Psychosocial perspective in the explanation of patients' drug taking behavior. *Soc Sci Med.* 1988;27:277–85.
22. Gupchup GV, Marfatia AA, Bartley M, et al. Intention to use herbal medicines among older outpatients. *J Soc Adm Pharm.* 2003;20;249–56.
23. Berger BA, Grimley D. Pharmacists' readiness for rendering pharmaceutical care. *J Am Pharm Assoc.* 1997;NS37:535–42.
24. Hudmon KS, Berger BA. Pharmacy applications of the transtheoretical model in smoking cessation. *Am J Health Syst Pharm.* 1995;52:282–7.
25. Prochaska J, DiClemente C, Norcross J. In search of how people change: applications to addictive behaviors. *Am J Psychol.* 1992;47:1102–14.

Additional Readings

Berger BA, Hudmon KS. Readiness for change: implications for patient care. *J Am Pharm Assoc.* 1997;NS37:321–9.
Chinburapa V, Larson LN. Explaining the intended use of nonprescription analgesics: test of the Fishbein Behavioral Intention Model. *J Pharm Mark Manage.* 1990;5(2);3–25.
Ficke DL, Farris KB. Use of the transtheoretical model in the medication use process. *Ann Pharmacother.* 2005;39:1325–30
Fincham JE, Wertheimer AI. Using the health belief model to predict initial drug therapy defaulting. *Soc Sci Med.* 1985;20:101–5.
Gaither CA, Bagozzi RP, Ascione FJ, et al. The determinants of physician attitudes and subjective norms toward drug information sources: modification and test of the theory of reasoned action. *Pharm Res.* 1997;14:1298–1308.
Ganther JM, Kreling DH. Consumer perceptions of risk and required cost savings for generic prescription drugs. *J Am Pharm Assoc.* 2000;40:378–83.
Grabenstein JD, Guess HA, Hartzema AG, et al. Attitudinal factors among adult prescription recipients associated with choice of where to be vaccinated. *J Clin Epidemiol.* 2002;55:279–84.
Johnson SS, Grimley DM, Prochaska JO. Prediction of adherence using the transtheoretical model: implications for pharmacy care practice. *J Soc Adm Pharm.* 1998;15(3):135–48.
Orensky IA, Holdford DA. Predictors of noncompliance with warfarin therapy in an outpatient anticoagulation clinic. *Pharmacotherapy.* 2005;25:1801–8.
Rees D. Feelings outweigh facts. *Pharm Exec.* 2006;2:S28–S33.

Exercises and Questions

1. What economic, social, and personal influences affected your decision to become a pharmacist? What influences will determine your career choices?
2. Identify decisions in health care that you consider risky and not risky. How might perceptions of risk affect how patients progress through each stage of the consumer decision-making model in Figure 6-2?
3. Discuss the different types of risk faced by patients who are seeking treatment for migraine headaches.
4. Name several pharmaceutical products. Classify them into what you perceive to be high and low involvement categories. How might you counsel patients differently about high versus low involvement products?
5. In general terms, discuss the value of consumer behavior models. How can a pharmacist use them to better influence patient behavior?

Activities

1. Select a significant purchase you have made and describe both your thoughts and your actions as you proceeded through each of the decision-making steps of (a) need recognition, (b) information search, (c) evaluation of alternatives, (d) consumption, and (e) postpurchase evaluation.
2. Select one of the following health behavior models and describe how pharmacists can use it to help patients take their medications correctly.
   a. Health belief model.
   b. Theory of reasoned action/theory of planned behavior.
   c. Transtheoretical model.

CONSUMERS' EVALUATION OF SERVICE

The young pharmacist, Scott, could not understand what made patients tick. Here he was, the most clinically competent employee in the pharmacy. But when patients came to the pharmacy, they always asked for Julius. Julius was an older pharmacist who was OK but not nearly as good as Scott. Julius would waste time chatting with patients about family members, the weather, and other trivial issues. He was not especially quick, but he seemed to make patients happy. When Scott dealt with patients, he was quick and professional. He always counseled the patients, whether or not they wanted counseling. Still, the patients continued to ask for Julius.

FIGURE 7-1   Factors affecting customer satisfaction.

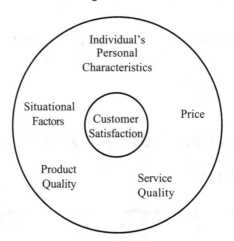

This chapter discusses how consumers evaluate services—pharmacist services in particular. It explains what determines satisfaction and perceptions of service quality. Important dimensions of service and their impact on overall assessments of service are also discussed. Finally, the chapter describes the link between patient perceptions of service and patient behavior.

SATISFACTION

In Chapter 6, satisfaction was described as an important and desired outcome of pharmacy services. Satisfaction results when a consumer evaluates a purchase he or she has made and concludes that the product or service meets or exceeds expectations.[1] When a product or service fails to meet expectations, dissatisfaction results.

Various factors contribute to satisfaction or dissatisfaction with pharmacy service experiences (Figure 7-1). Satisfaction with a pharmacy visit may be influenced by the responsiveness of the pharmacist to the needs of the patient (i.e., service quality), perceptions of how the drug worked (i.e., product quality), and the price paid (i.e., value).

Satisfaction is also influenced by factors beyond the marketer's control. Both the situation in which the service is provided and the characteristics of the person assessing the service affect satisfaction. The weather or traffic on the way to the pharmacy can influence a patient's evaluation, as can personal factors like fatigue or irritability.

FIGURE 7-2 Results of comparing perceived service performance with expectations.

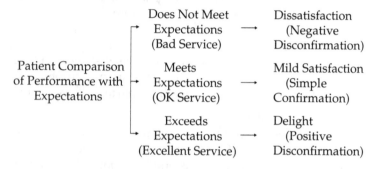

The comparison of performance with expectations is called the process of expectancy disconfirmation (Figure 7-2).[2] Disconfirmation of expectations can be positive or negative. *Negative disconfirmation* occurs when performance does not meet expectations; the consumer is dissatisfied. When performance meets expectations, *confirmation* occurs; the consumer is either mildly satisfied or not dissatisfied. *Positive disconfirmation* occurs when performance exceeds expectations; the consumer is satisfied. "Customer delight"[3] occurs when the consumer is extremely satisfied as a result of some unexpected, pleasant surprise (e.g., a pharmacist who goes out of the way to help solve a patient problem).

As an example of disconfirmation, consider a woman who visits a pharmacy with her 7-year-old daughter to fill a prescription for the child's ear infection. In the past, the girl has been very finicky about taking medications. Administering each dose has been a major battle between the mother and the child. In addition, the mother is anxious about the girl's health, and the illness has disrupted the whole family's daily routine.

If the pharmacist fills the prescription quickly and accurately, the mother's expectations are met and she is mildly satisfied with the service. The mother's anxiety about her finicky child has not been resolved, but her minimal expectation of receiving the drug in a timely manner has been met. If the mother's minimal expectation is not met (e.g., the pharmacist makes the mother wait too long or is unintentionally rude), negative disconfirmation occurs and the mother is dissatisfied.

But the pharmacist does more than what is minimally expected. He speaks directly to the girl in a pleasant and serious manner. Crouching down to her eye level, he tells the girl about the antibiotic and the importance of taking it. The girl is allowed to choose from several flavorings (bubblegum, grape, cherry). The pharmacist adds the girl's choice (bubblegum) and water to the powdered drug and then asks the girl to help shake the ingredients in the bottle. The pharmacist tells the girl that it is her responsibility to shake the medicine before every dose; otherwise, the medicine will not work. With great seriousness and commitment, the girl shakes the bottle and promises to follow the pharmacist's directions. The mother is delighted, because she has just seen a pharmacist persuade her finicky child to take the medication. The pharmacy has just gained a loyal customer, because the pharmacist went out of the way to help.

Consumer satisfaction is important to marketers and service providers for several reasons. Satisfaction with businesses has been shown to increase repeat purchasing intentions and behaviors.[4–7] Consumers who are satisfied are more likely to say good things to friends and family members and less likely to complain to them.[5] Positive word of mouth can often be more effective in attracting new customers than most forms of advertising and promotion.[8]

Furthermore, businesses that continually satisfy customers with quality services are more profitable, on average. Satisfaction has been associated with increased market share, the ability to charge customers higher prices, higher return on investment, and profitability.[7,9]

EXPECTATIONS

It is clear from the previous discussion that expectations about service delivery and outcome are an important aspect of satisfaction. Zeithaml and Bitner[10] state that expectations are a blend of desires for what a service can be and what it should be (i.e., what would be ideal and what is necessary).

Consumers' evaluation of services is affected by their expectations about performance. Consumers who have low expectations are easy to please, and those with high expectations are more likely to be disappointed. Performance can be categorized as equitable, ideal, or expected.[11] Equitable performance refers to expectations of what *should* be received; it is what consumers perceive as a fair performance level. Ideal performance refers to expectations of the best performance possible. Expected performance refers to what performance is likely to be.

Consumer expectations of services have upper and lower boundaries: minimally acceptable and most desired[10] (i.e., adequate for minimal satisfaction, and likely to produce customer delight, respectively). Services that fall between minimally acceptable and most desired are in the zone of tolerance[12] (Figure 7-3). Service in the zone of tolerance is perceived as

FIGURE 7-3 Zone of tolerance for services. (Compiled from reference 12.)

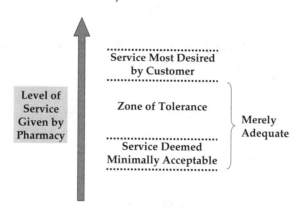

neither excellent nor bad. It is merely adequate and causes only mild satisfaction. Services that consistently fall within the zone of tolerance neither attract customers nor drive them away.

Merely adequate services provide no competitive advantage to businesses. When service is only adequate, competitive advantage must come from other sources, such as merchandise, location, price, or other elements of the marketing mix.

Pharmacists who merely meet patient expectations provide the minimum performance necessary to satisfy patients. Meeting expectations is fine in an environment without competition. It generates mildly positive feelings about the pharmacist and keeps the patient loyal—as long as no competitor offers anything better.

PERCEIVED VALUE AND SERVICE QUALITY

Also related to consumers' perceptions of service are perceived value and service quality. Perceived value is the consumer's overall assessment of utility, based on comparing what is received with what was spent in dollars, time, and effort.[10] In other words, value refers to a consumer's perception of the tradeoff between benefits and costs. A patient's perception of the value of pharmacy services depends on the quality of those services, the benefits resulting from that quality, and the amount of money, time, and effort spent in receiving those benefits. Value will be discussed in more detail in Chapter 12, on pricing.

Service quality refers to customer perceptions of the quality of services over time. It is closely related to, yet distinct from, satisfaction.[13] Satisfaction refers to customer perceptions not only of the quality of services but also of products, price, and other non-service-related factors. Satisfaction can relate to a short-term, transaction-specific evaluation[13] or, like service quality, to a long-term perception of performance over time.[14]

SERVICE ELEMENTS ASSESSED BY CONSUMERS

Search and Nonsearch Qualities

Some services can be difficult to assess. When you go to an auto mechanic, it is difficult to know whether the mechanic performed all the services he claims to have performed. In most cases, you have to take the mechanic's word that he replaced a part or changed a fluid.

Similarly, the quality of a pharmacist's work in filling a prescription can be difficult to assess, because patients cannot evaluate factors such as the accuracy of record keeping or the clinical expertise of the pharmacist. Some aspects of pharmacy service can be evaluated only after consumption (e.g., a pharmacist's recommendation for a nonprescription headache medication).

Attributes that a consumer can identify and evaluate before choosing or consuming a service are said to have *search qualities*.[15] A pharmacy's location has search qualities because the consumer can evaluate it by finding it on a map or driving past it. Attributes that cannot be evaluated before purchase or use are said to have *nonsearch qualities*; pain relief from a recommended drug and the friendliness of pharmacy personnel are examples.

Nonsearch qualities are further classified into experience and credence subcategories (Table 7-1).[16] *Experience qualities* can be evaluated during or after consumption. Service can be experienced as friendly or fast while it is taking place. A drug recommendation for relief of pain or allergic

TABLE 7-1   Service Qualities and Consumers' Ability to Assess Them

Description	Definition	Examples
Search qualities	Attributes that can be identified and evaluated prior to choice or consumption	Cleanliness Price Convenience
Nonsearch (experience) qualities	Attributes that can be evaluated during or after consumption only	Speed of service Reliability and friendliness of service personnel Responsiveness to needs
Nonsearch (credence) qualities	Attributes that cannot be evaluated even after consumption	Clinical competence of pharmacists Therapeutic knowledge

Source: Reference 16.

symptoms can be evaluated after the medication is used. *Credence qualities,* on the other hand, cannot be meaningfully evaluated even after an experience. Most technical services provided by pharmacists, such as therapeutic drug monitoring, have credence quali-

> *Patients tend to rate their pharmacists on the basis of their social interactions rather than their technical skills.*

ties, because patients do not have the knowledge or expertise to evaluate the services even after receiving them. Many medications must be used for long periods of time before their effects can be seen, and even then it may be uncertain whether the patient's health outcome was the result of a particular therapy.

In general, medical services have credence qualities and are therefore difficult to assess. Like all services, they are intangible, inconsistent, and inseparable. Moreover, the practice of medicine is complex and requires substantial training and education. Most patients feel uncomfortable judging the more technical aspects of medical care.

For these reasons, patients are likely to assess health care services on the basis of search and experience qualities.[17,18] Patient satisfaction with physician visits is likely to be determined more by the amount of time the physician spends with the patient (experience) than by the technical aspects of care. In choosing pharmacies, patients rely on search (e.g., convenience) and experience (e.g., speedy and friendly service) characteristics.[19,20]

Technical and Functional Quality

Gronroos[21] states that the quality of services has both technical and functional components. *Technical quality* refers to the end result of services (i.e., outcomes). Elements of pharmacist services that affect technical quality are those activities that result in receiving the right drug and maximizing the appropriateness of drug use (e.g., reviewing the patient medication profile, therapeutic monitoring, and counseling). *Functional quality* refers to the process in which services are provided (e.g., responsive, reliable).

Patients judge pharmacy service quality on the basis of their perceptions of both the technical and functional components,[22] and functional quality plays a greater role. Although a positive outcome of pharmacy service is always desired, patients tend to rate their pharmacists on the basis of their social interactions rather than their technical skills. Ried et al.[23] found that patient satisfaction was influenced more by a pharmacist's prompt personal attention to requests, willingness to spend time, and friendliness than by perceptions of the pharmacist's ability to control the patient's asthma. Holdford and Schulz[22] also found that functional quality in a dispensing situation has greater impact than technical quality on patient perceptions of pharmacy services.

Patients do not have the expertise or information necessary to evaluate the technical quality of health care. Instead, they consider how personable a pharmacist is or how neatly she is dressed. In fact, a technically competent pharmacist with poor interpersonal skills may be rated lower by patients than a less competent pharmacist with good interpersonal capabilities.

Dimensions of Service

Marketers refer to 10 generic dimensions that are important in consumers' evaluation of service (Table 7-2).[24] These dimensions primarily address functional quality.

Although any of the 10 dimensions can determine a consumer's judgment of service, some dimensions are more important than others. Reliability is considered the most important driver of overall perception of services.[13,25] Reliability addresses the question, "Are services provided accurately and dependably?" It also indirectly relates to other service dimensions such as credibility (i.e., Will the pharmacist keep his promises?) and competence (i.e., Is the pharmacist competent to provide services without mistakes?).

Reliability is a core element of value provided by pharmacists. A pharmacist's work is expected to be error free; otherwise, a patient could be injured or even killed. Reliability is also the foundation for credibility and trust. A pharmacist who is not dependable or cannot be expected to keep promises will not be able to maintain the trust of customers.

The second most important dimension driving consumers' evaluation of service is responsiveness.[13,25] Responsiveness encompasses both willingness and capability to respond to customers in a timely manner. A responsive pharmacist is attentive to patients' requests for assistance, questions about the location of pharmacy merchandise, and complaints about services. Even when a pharmacist cannot solve a patient's problem, it is essential that the pharmacist be perceived as willing to do so. Responsiveness also refers to the perceived speed of service. A patient who has to wait for prescriptions or counseling about medications typically rates responsiveness as low.

Other dimensions of service quality can determine whether a consumer will patronize a business. Credibility is essential in health care.

TABLE 7-2 Dimensions of Service Quality

Tangibles: The appearance of physical facilities and personnel. The tools or equipment used to provide the service. Written information provided as part of the service.

Reliability: Performing the service correctly the first time. Honoring promises through accurate billing, precise record keeping, and performance of the service when promised.

Responsiveness: Willingness and ability to provide prompt service. Involves timeliness of service.

Communication: Explaining service to customers in language they can understand. Involves explaining the service itself, describing how much it will cost, explaining the tradeoffs between service and cost, and assuring the customer that the problem will be resolved.

Credibility: Trustworthiness, believability, and honesty of customer-contact personnel and company.

Security: Freedom from danger, risk, and doubt. Involves physical safety (e.g., Will following the pharmacist's directions cause me harm?), financial security (e.g., Will I be able to pay for my drugs?), and confidentiality of transactions (e.g., Will the other customers hear about my physical ailments?).

Competence: Customer-contact personnel's possession of the required skills and knowledge to perform the service.

Understanding/knowing the customer: Involves learning a customer's specific requirements, providing individualized attention, and recognizing a regular customer.

Access: Involves approachability and ease of contact. Includes accessibility by telephone, convenient operating hours and location, and reasonable waiting time for service.

Courtesy: Politeness, respect, consideration, and friendliness of customer-contact personnel. Includes clean and neat appearance of customer-contact personnel.

Source: Reference 24.

Pharmacists make recommendations that affect a patient's health and daily activities. Those recommendations must inspire patients' trust and confidence. Communication is necessary to help patients understand how to take their medications and to clear up misunderstandings about issues such as pricing. The risk associated with prescription drugs makes security an important dimension. Even the physical appearance of facilities and personnel (*tangibles*) sends a message of competence and quality to patients.

The relative importance of individual dimensions in the evaluation of a service experience depends in part on the consumer and the circumstances of the visit. A pharmacy's appearance may be important for someone who is shopping for birthday cards but irrelevant for a quick visit to purchase soda or snacks.

To maximize patient assessments of service quality, pharmacists should focus on being reliable first and responsive second. This means putting a system in place in which errors do not occur, service is timely, and employees care about serving the patient. When these dimensions of service are maintained at a consistently high level, pharmacists can work on the other dimensions of service.

MAINTAINING CUSTOMER LOYALTY

Customers' satisfaction and perception of service quality are important because they relate to measures of business performance, including profitability. Consumer perceptions of service are frequently used as a proxy measure for consumer behavior and business profitability.

One problem with using satisfaction as the sole outcome measure of services is that the link between satisfaction and patronage tends to be weak and inconsistent. Even when satisfied, consumers often switch to other service providers. Research shows that between 65% and 85% of consumers who report being satisfied or very satisfied with their former service provider will switch to other providers.[26] Even consumers who are considered loyal continue to do business with other providers.[27,28] This suggests that consumer satisfaction alone may be a poor predictor of profitability.

Thus, when given freedom of choice, a satisfied patient of a community pharmacy may decide to visit a competing pharmacy just out of curiosity or because of a discount on a transferred prescription. Even when content, people may investigate other providers for better service and price offers, particularly if there is no perception of risk or hassle involved.[29]

Restrictions on the freedom to choose pharmacies can further cloud the link between satisfaction and patronage. When a pharmacy benefit manager restricts patients to a limited network of pharmacies, patients may be dissatisfied with the network pharmacies but continue to use them to avoid paying for their drugs out of pocket. In rural areas, dissatisfied patients may continue to patronize a pharmacy if competing pharmacies are too far away. In these cases, satisfaction may have little relationship to patient patronage and thus profitability.

Businesses have begun to emphasize the importance of customer loyalty, as well as satisfaction. Customer loyalty is defined as continual patronage of a service provider, and it is claimed to be the single most important determinant of long-term financial performance.[30] Loyal customers lead to increased profitability and productivity because they are more likely to repurchase goods and services and to repurchase in greater quantity, and they cost less to retain.[7,30-32]

> *Improvements in consumer satisfaction are not necessarily associated with equivalent changes in consumer loyalty.*

Customer loyalty involves positive feelings toward an organization as well as ongoing patronage.[30,32] Thus, loyalty has both an affective and a behavioral component. When consumers speak highly of a business or express a preference over competitors, this is *affective loyalty*. People who are delighted with a business express affective loyalty. When consumers increase purchases of goods and services or willingly pay a premium price, this is *behavioral loyalty*. Consumers who have high levels of affective loyalty are also likely to demonstrate high levels of behavioral loyalty.[30,32]

Satisfaction and Behavioral Loyalty

The relationship between consumer satisfaction and behavioral loyalty often is not linear. Improvements in consumer satisfaction are not necessarily associated with equivalent changes in consumer loyalty.

The relationship between satisfaction and behavioral loyalty depends in part on a consumer's ability to freely move from one service provider to another.[31,33] If consumers are free to choose, dissatisfaction will lead to decreased loyalty. But consumers' ability to respond to dissatisfaction may be restricted by a lack of competitors or by contractual limitations of prescription insurance plans. Thus, in noncompetitive environments, such as rural areas underserved by pharmacists, locales where patients do not have freedom of pharmacy choice because of managed care restrictions, and communities where a pharmacy may be the only provider offering a unique, highly desired service, there is much less sensitivity to changes in patient satisfaction. Only when consumers become extremely dissatisfied will substantial defections to competitors occur.

In noncompetitive environments, relationships with a business may be based on some barrier to leaving that relationship, not on a continued desire to maintain the relationship. Dissatisfied consumers maintain a relationship only as long as they must. Once the barriers that prevent free choice are removed, the consumer very likely will leave that service provider.

Effect of Dissatisfaction

Negative experiences with pharmacy service are likely to have a greater impact on overall patient satisfaction than positive service experiences. Pro-

> *Consumers pay more attention to bad service than to good service.*

viding excellent service is important in exceeding patient expectations, but it is more important not to dissatisfy patients with poor service experiences.[34,35] When a prescription is filled 10 minutes faster than promised or expected, this has a positive but limited effect on overall patient satisfaction. Waiting 10 minutes longer than expected for a prescription is likely to have a disproportionately greater negative effect on overall satisfaction.

The reason is that consumers pay more attention to bad service than to good service and are more likely to remember bad service experiences.[36] Consumers expect to receive good service in most cases. If prescriptions are dispensed correctly, patients will only be "not dissatisfied," because error-free dispensing is taken for granted. But when expectations of good service are not met, patients may feel unfairly treated and take action in response.

That action might include discontinuing business with the service provider or complaining to others. Consumers are more likely to complain to others about bad service than to make positive comments about good service. Consumers tell an average of 5 other people when they receive good service, whereas they tell 9 to 11 others when they receive bad service.[31] Because consumers attach more significance to negative service experiences, a highly satisfied consumer can quickly become a highly dissatisfied consumer.

IMPROVING PATIENT PERCEPTIONS OF SERVICE

Assessing Perceptions of Service

There are many ways for pharmacists to assess patient perceptions of service.[37,38] They differ in complexity, cost, and the degree to which they inconvenience the patient. Table 7-3 lists common assessment methods. To maximize the use of these methods, pharmacists may want to consult experienced researchers.

Observation

The easiest assessment method is observation. Observing the reactions of patients in a pharmacy can suggest better ways to provide service. One business has made a science of observing how people behave while

TABLE 7-3 Methods of Assessing Patient Perceptions of Pharmacy Services

Method	Purpose
Observation	Observing patient interactions with pharmacists and technicians can identify service problems. Observation can identify unproductive practices, length of time spent in various activities, and customer responses.
Employee feedback	Employees know many of the problems within service systems and can suggest solutions. They can also assess the quality of internal marketing initiatives. Employee feedback should be solicited with any service venture.
Patient complaints	Patient complaints can help identify which aspects of service are most irritating. Complaints may indicate just the tip of the iceberg and reveal a serious service problem. Service recovery strategies should be developed to deal with complaints.
Patient interviews	Patients can be interviewed formally or casually about their assessments of pharmacist services. Most good pharmacists ask patients how they are doing and how they can improve.
Patient surveys	Surveys can solicit patient feedback about service while experiences are still fresh in the patient's mind. The shorter and more accessible the survey, the better.
Critical incident surveys	Critical incident surveys are designed to identify particularly good and bad services. Patients are asked to describe the details of service incidents that stand out in their minds (e.g., "Describe a particularly good or bad experience you had with a pharmacist").
Focus groups	Focus groups are gatherings of patients who are invited to discuss issues of importance. They can be used to solicit quick, informal insight into service problems.
Mystery (secret) shoppers	Mystery shoppers are individuals paid to shop at a pharmacy in order to systematically assess a checklist of service standards. This method can be used to identify strengths and weaknesses of the service system.
Service audits	Service audits are systematic assessments of the entire service system. They are described in Chapter 5.
Sales figures	Sales figures are the ultimate measure of patient satisfaction. Patient perceptions of service should be linked to total sales, repeat sales, and other sales figures to identify which measures are most predictive of sales.

they shop.[39] The firm, Envirosell, measures and records the actions of customers as they shop. Employees record what shoppers look at, touch, and do from the moment they enter a business to the time they leave. They measure how long people spend in different activities and how they move throughout stores while they shop.

Envirosell has found that, in many businesses, promotional and directional signs face the direction opposite that in which people circulate through the store. Therefore, it is common for customers to have trouble finding merchandise.

Also, nonprescription drug sections that are located in busy areas of pharmacies are often less profitable than those located in quiet sections. That is because buyers of nonprescription products prefer to make their purchase decisions in private.

Immediately inside the doorway of every business is a transition zone, where customers become accustomed to the store lighting and layout. The size of the zone varies for each business, and merchandise displays within the zone tend to be ignored and bypassed. The lesson for marketers is to move merchandise displays further inside the store.

People who have their hands free will buy more. Keeping shopping bags and carts easily accessible can increase purchases.

Finally, Envirosell found that customers do not purchase as much from a display that is located in a crowded aisle. Women, in particular, do not like to be brushed or touched from behind as people move past them. Even if the display has products of interest, shoppers will avoid it.

Employee Feedback

Many businesses conduct employee satisfaction surveys, because satisfied employees are more likely to provide good service. In addition to questions about overall satisfaction with compensation and working conditions, employees should be asked what aspects of the organization (e.g., policies, structural problems) inhibit their ability to serve the customer.

Patient Feedback

Patient feedback can be collected in many ways. Patient complaints can be solicited through toll-free telephone numbers, patient comment cards, or service departments. Patient interviews can be conducted during service provision or in a more formal setting, such as a patient counseling area. Patient surveys and critical incident reports can be completed in person or by mail, telephone, or Internet. Focus groups can be conducted anywhere a pharmacist can get people to meet, such as in a public building, a marketing research facility, or even the pharmacy itself. The choice of technique depends on the purpose of the feedback, the budget, and the available time.

> *The key to making patient feedback pay off is to develop a tracking system that permits analysis and action.*

The key to making patient feedback pay off is to develop a tracking system that permits analysis and action. Patient responses that are simply filed away cannot be used to improve service. Furthermore, to obtain usable recommendations for improving service, the right questions need to be asked, in a way that effectively elicits patient comments.

Mystery Shoppers

Mystery, or secret, shoppers are sometimes used to supplement patient feedback. They provide analysis of specific service features that patient feedback may overlook. A mystery shopper who visits a pharmacy typically has a checklist for assessing aspects of service such as whether the pharmacist greeted the patient, offered to counsel about the medications, was friendly and helpful, checked the patient profile, and completed other required tasks. Most patients are not able to assess the service experience as critically or in as much detail as trained and observant mystery shoppers can.

Measuring Loyalty

Loyalty should be measured, since it is an important indicator of profitability. Measures of loyalty include intention to repurchase, actual repurchase, and positive word-of-mouth recommendations.[30]

It is easy and convenient to ask consumers about intentions to repurchase a product or service. (Measuring intention to repurchase is based on the theories of reasoned action and planned behavior, described in Chapter 6.) Intention-to-repurchase measures are strong indicators of future behavior, but they generally overstate the probability of repurchase.[30] People who report that they intend to purchase do not always do so. Usually this overstatement is not a significant problem, because the extent of overstatement is consistent. Adjustments can be made to correct for the overstatement, resulting in relatively accurate predictions.[30]

Sales data provide information about actual repurchase behavior, including how recently, how frequently, and how long repurchases have occurred and the amounts of these purchases.[30,33] These measurements can be used to determine change resulting from marketing interventions. The data are easy to gather from computer databases. In pharmacy firms, repurchase data might include the percentage of patients who refill prescriptions or transfer prescriptions to other pharmacies.

Consumer referrals and positive word-of-mouth recommendations are associated with short-term and long-term judgments about purchasing behavior.[30] Such referrals and recommendations indicate the strength of feelings about services (i.e., affective loyalty); they are less directly linked to actual purchase behavior. When all forms of loyalty measures are used together, they can provide a comprehensive picture of consumer loyalty and can supplement satisfaction data.

Prioritizing Service Quality Initiatives

Pharmacists have limited resources to improve the quality of their services, so they need to select marketing approaches that optimize patient loyalty. It often pays for pharmacists to focus on service deficiencies to reduce dissatisfaction, rather than trying to increase satisfaction. To reduce the number of patients dissatisfied with a pharmacy organization, several strategies can be used.[10,27,40]

First, target patients who can be best satisfied by the pharmacy. Some individuals become dissatisfied with services not through the fault of the program, but because they are just a poor match for what the program offers. Patient selection is critical for ensuring that patient expectations match the services being provided.

Also, educate patients about what to expect. When expectations are unreasonable, open communication with the patient can sometimes adjust expectations.

Prevent service-related failures from occurring in the first place. This requires a service system that continually seeks to root out causes of failure and correct them.

Practice service recovery once a service failure has occurred. Pharmacies need to have a plan in place for use when failures occur.

SUMMARY

Patients base their evaluations of pharmacy services on a complex mix of expectations and perceptions. Positive perceptions are associated with patient loyalty, positive word-of-mouth recommendations, and profitability.

Pharmacists who want to maximize their impact on patient perceptions should focus on specific aspects of their services. They should attempt to make their service as reliable and responsive as possible, and to minimize negative service experiences. Finally, pharmacists should monitor patient perceptions of service to identify ways of improving the services they provide.

References

1. Hunt KH. Consumer satisfaction, dissatisfaction, and complaining behavior. *J Soc Issues.* 1991;47(1):109–10.
2. Oliver RL. A cognitive model of the antecedents and consequences of satisfaction decisions. *J Mark Res.* 1980;17:460–9.
3. Oliver RL, Rust RT, Varki S. Customer delight: foundations, findings, and managerial insight. *J Retailing.* 1997;73:311–36.
4. Anderson EW, Fornell C, Lehmann DR. Customer satisfaction, market share, and profitability—findings from Sweden. *J Mark.* 1994;58:53–66.
5. Bearden WO, Teel JE. Selected determinants of consumer satisfaction and complaint reports. *J Mark Res.* February 1983;6:21–8.
6. Bolton RN, Drew JH. A multistage model of customers' assessments of service quality and value. *J Consum Res.* 1991;17:375–84.
7. Zeithaml VA, Berry LL, Parasuraman A. The behavioral consequences of service quality. *J Mark.* 1996;60:31–46.
8. Gladwell M. *The Tipping Point.* New York: Little, Brown and Co; 2000.
9. Rust RT, Zahorik AJ, Keiningham TL. Return on quality (ROQ)—making service quality financially accountable. *J Mark.* 1995;59:58–70.
10. Zeithaml VA, Bitner M. *Services Marketing.* New York: McGraw-Hill Co Inc; 1996.
11. Engel JF, Blackwell RD, Miniard PW. *Consumer Behavior.* Fort Worth, Tex: Dryden Press; 1993.
12. Zeithaml V, Berry LL, Parasuraman A. The nature and determinants of customer expectations of service. *J Acad Mark Sci.* 1993;21(1):1–12.
13. Parasuraman A, Zeithaml V, Berry L. SERVQUAL: a multi item scale for measuring consumer perception of service quality. *J Retailing.* 1988;64: 12–40.
14. Bitner MJ, Hubbert AR. Encounter satisfaction vs. overall satisfaction vs. quality: the customer's voice. In: Rust RT, Oliver RL, eds. *Service Quality: New Directions in Theory and Practice.* Newbury Park, Calif: Sage; 1993: 71–93.
15. Nelson P. Information and consumer behavior. *J Polit Econ.* 1970;78:311–29.
16. Darby MR, Karni E. Free competition and the optimal amount of fraud. *J Law Econ.* 1973;16:67–86.
17. Lynch J, Schuler D. Consumer evaluation of the quality of hospital services from an economics of information perspective. *J Health Care Mark.* 1990;10:16–22.
18. Murray KB. Health care service decision influences: an exploratory investigation of search and nonsearch criteria for professionals and patients. *J Health Care Mark.* 1992;12:24–38.

19. Roller K. Convenience dominates when choosing a pharmacy. *Drug Store News.* 1999;221(14):17.

20. Wiederholt JB. Development of an instrument to measure evaluative criteria that patients use in selecting a pharmacy for obtaining prescription drugs. *J Pharm Mark Manage.* 1987;1:35–59.

21. Gronroos C. *Service Management and Marketing.* Lexington, Mass: Lexington Books; 1990.

22. Holdford D, Schulz R. Effect of technical and functional quality on patient perceptions of pharmaceutical service quality. *Pharm Res.* 1999;16: 1344–51.

23. Ried LD, Wang F, Young H, et al. Patients' satisfaction and their perception of the pharmacist. *J Am Pharm Assoc.* 1999;39:835–42.

24. Parasuraman A, Zeithaml V, Berry L. A conceptual model of service quality and its implications for future research. *J Mark.* 1985;49:41–50.

25. Parasuraman A, Zeithaml V, Berry L. Refinement and reassessment of the SERVQUAL scale. *J Retailing.* 1991;67:420–50.

26. Reichheld FF. Loyalty-based management. *Harv Bus Rev.* 1993;71:64–73.

27. Griffin J. *Customer Loyalty: How to Earn It. How to Keep It.* San Francisco: Jossey-Bass Publishers; 1995.

28. O'Malley L. Can loyalty schemes really build loyalty? *Mark Intell Plann.* 1998;16:47–55.

29. Dowling GR, Uncles M. Do customer loyalty programs really work? *Sloan Manage Rev.* 1997;38:71–92.

30. Jones TO, Sasser WE. Why satisfied customers defect. *Harv Bus Rev.* 1995; 73:88–99.

31. Heskett JL, Sasser ED, Schlesinger LA. *The Service Profit Chain.* New York: The Free Press; 1997.

32. Reichheld FF. Learning from customer defections. *Harv Bus Rev.* 1996;74: 56–69.

33. Oliva TA, Oliver RL, MacMillan IC. A catastrophe model for developing service satisfaction strategies. *J Mark.* 1992;56:83–95.

34. Mittal V, Ross WT, Baldasare PM. The asymmetric impact of negative and positive attribute-level performance on overall satisfaction and repurchase intentions. *J Mark.* 1998;62:33–47.

35. Mittal V, Lassar WM. Why do customers switch? The dynamics of satisfaction versus loyalty. *J Serv Mark.* 1998;12:177–94.

36. Mittal V, Baldasare PM. Eliminate the negative: managers should optimize rather than maximize performance to enhance patient satisfaction. *J Health Care Mark.* 1996;16:24–7.

37. Berry LL, Parasuraman A. Listening to the customer—the concept of a service quality information system. *Sloan Manage Rev.* 1997;38:65–76.

38. Ford RC, Bach SA, Fottler MD. Methods of measuring patient satisfaction in health care organizations. *Health Care Manage Rev.* 1997;22:74–89.

39. Underhill P. *Why We Buy: The Science of Shopping.* New York: Simon and Schuster; 1999.

40. Heskett JL, Jones TO, Loveman GW, et al. Putting the service-profit chain to work. *Harv Bus Rev.* 1994;72:164–74.

Additional Readings

Bentley JP, Stroup LJ, Wilkin NE, et al. Patient evaluations of pharmacist performance with variations in attire and communication levels. *J Am Pharm Assoc.* 2005;45:600–7.

Kucukarslan S. Identifying patient needs in the context of the medication use situation. *J Am Pharm Assoc.* 1998;38:440–5.

Nau DP, Erickson SR. Medication safety: patients' experiences, beliefs, and behaviors. *J Am Pharm Assoc.* 2005;45:452–7.

Nau DP, Ried LD, Lipowski EE, et al. Patients' perceptions of the benefits of pharmaceutical care. *J Am Pharm Assoc.* 2000;40:36–40.

Schommer JC, Kucukarslan SN. Measuring patient satisfaction with pharmaceutical services. *Am J Health Syst Pharm.* 1997;54:2721–32.

Yang Z, Peterson RT, Huang L. Taking the pulse of Internet pharmacies. *Mark Health Serv.* 2001;21(2):4–10.

Exercises and Questions

1. Discuss the differences between confirmation, negative disconfirmation, and positive disconfirmation.

2. Is it necessary for patients to be satisfied with their health care? Should pharmacists attempt to achieve 100% patient satisfaction? Explain your answer.

3. How might patient expectations influence perceptions of pharmacist performance? What determines patient expectations of pharmacist services? In what situations might pharmacists want to lower patient expectations?

4. Describe the relationship between patient satisfaction and loyalty to the pharmacy.

5. Which of the 10 dimensions of service quality are most important in patients' overall perception of pharmacist services? In your opinion, which ones are least important?

6. How might patients and pharmacists differ in their perceptions of the quality of pharmacy services? Who would be the most critical of the services, and why?

7. Suggest examples of search, experience, and credence qualities for pharmacy education (the professors are service providers and the students are customers).

8. How does functional quality influence the technical quality of pharmacy services?

9. Discuss the relative merits of the methods listed in Table 7-3 for assessing patient perceptions of pharmacy services.

Activities

1. Develop a plan for assessing the quality of pharmacy services, using three methods of your choice from Table 7-3. Explain how the three methods differs from each other in the way they provide insights into patient perceptions of service.
2. Use the information from this chapter to develop a list of "Dos and Don'ts" for pharmacist services (e.g., Do always call customers by their names).
3. Working in groups, classify each journal entry from the Chapter 3 Activity according to the 10 service quality dimensions in Table 7-2. What dimensions were associated with the most negative service experiences? Positive service experiences?

PART IV

MARKETING STRATEGY

8

STRATEGIC MARKETING PLANNING

Objectives

After studying this chapter, the reader should be able to

- ❑ Describe the strategic planning process.
- ❑ Discuss the role of strategic marketing planning for pharmacists.
- ❑ Define the following terms associated with strategic planning: *mission statement, business plan, SWOT analysis, marketing goals and objectives, brand, commodity, brand awareness, brand image, brand equity.*
- ❑ Develop a strategic marketing plan for a pharmaceutical service or product.

Karen Wesley is a newly hired pharmacist who has been asked to plan and implement a diabetes clinic at an independent pharmacy. The pharmacy provides a broad range of merchandise, including complementary medicines, gourmet and international foods, and specialty gifts, for an upscale clientele. Clinical pharmacy services are a new and expanding offering for the independent. In 2 weeks, Karen will be expected to present a marketing plan to the owner that delineates the program design, clientele served, local competition, and promotional strategy. Karen wonders where to start.

This chapter describes the steps involved in strategic marketing planning. It discusses the application of this process to problems faced by pharmacists.

SETTING ORGANIZATIONAL STRATEGIES

A strategy is a plan for accomplishing a goal. In reference to business, a strategy is a plan for moving the business from where it is now to where it wants to be in the future. Strategic planning requires that firms develop a clear understanding of their present circumstances, identify where they want to be, and create a plan for getting there.

In most organizations, strategy comes from the top management. In a typical pharmacy organization, the chief executive works with others in leadership positions to set a strategic direction for the organization. In a large pharmacy chain, the chief executive officer consults with other top executives on strategies. In an independent pharmacy, the pharmacist owner consults with managers and key employees.

The extent of pharmacists' involvement in developing organizational strategies depends on their job responsibilities, the business they work for, and their desire to become involved in the business. Strategic planning is a key responsibility in some pharmacist positions; this is more likely as pharmacists rise further within an organization. In some pharmacy organizations, everyone is encouraged to be involved in strategic planning, including staff pharmacists and technicians. This is most common in businesses that use an empowerment approach to management, in which many managerial decisions are delegated to employees and the employees are encouraged to take responsibility for new business ideas. In such organizations, the only limitation to pharmacist participation in strategic planning is pharmacists' willingness to participate.

ROLE OF THE MISSION STATEMENT

A mission statement is a broad yet specific statement of an organization's purpose for existence and its future direction. The mission statement plays a critical role in strategic planning. All planning and strategies for future action originate (or should) from the mission of the organization (Figure 8-1).

FIGURE 8-1   Elements of a simple business plan.

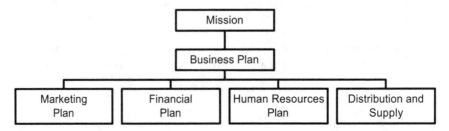

Most organizations have a formal mission statement that describes the customers served by the business, the needs the business fulfills for the customers, and the products and services provided to meet those needs. Here are the mission statements of three pharmacy organizations:

American Pharmacists Association: The American Pharmacists Association provides information, education, and advocacy to empower its members to improve medication use and advance patient care.[1]

Rite Aid: [Our mission is] to be a successful chain of friendly, neighborhood drugstores. Our knowledgeable, caring associates work together to provide a superior pharmacy experience, and offer everyday products and services that help our valued customers lead healthier, happier lives.[2]

Virginia Commonwealth University School of Pharmacy: The mission of the School of Pharmacy is to provide professional, graduate and postgraduate education, conduct pharmaceutical and biomedical research, and provide patient care and public service.[3]

Mission statements drive planning and decision-making. If an organization declares that a part of its mission is to improve patient health, then elements of the business plan should address how the company will do that. If business practices are inconsistent with the company mission, mission statements become hollow declarations with little meaning.

ROLE OF THE BUSINESS PLAN

From the mission comes the business plan (Figure 8-1), a blueprint on which all company decisions are based. The business plan contains goals and objectives for the operations of the organization. From those goals and objectives, strategies are formulated for finance, human resources, research and development, production, and marketing.

All plans and strategies developed and implemented throughout the organization, including marketing strategies, must be consistent with the organization's business plan. Pharmacists who propose the introduction of new pharmaceutical care services within a company must do so in a way that is in harmony with the mission of the company and the other functions of the organization. If the primary mission of the company is to dispense drugs cheaply without consideration of the health of patients, then pharmaceutical care services may conflict with the mission. However, if health care is a prominent feature of the mission, then pharmaceutical care services can be supported as part of the organization's purpose.

Marketing is but one operational area of a company that helps determine its success (Figure 8-1). All operational areas are equally important to the success or failure of a business. An organization that excels in marketing can fail if it does a poor job of controlling its finances. A company whose human resources operations cannot attract and keep the best employees will be unable to compete against companies that can. It is crucial that marketing strategy be integrated with the other functions of the organization.

DEVELOPING THE STRATEGIC MARKETING PLAN

Once the mission statement and business plan are established, plans can be made for marketing and other elements of the business. Strategic marketing planning consists of the following steps:

- Analyzing the market for opportunities and threats,
- Assessing the fit of one's mission, resources, and capabilities to the market environment,
- Choosing a course of action based on these analyses, and
- Assessing the success of the plan.

These steps may appear to be common sense, but pharmacists are typically not very good at strategic planning. Studies indicate that many pharmacy owners and managers do not conduct strategic planning, have little knowledge of the process, or do not consider it a priority in their practice.[4,5] This is surprising, because strategic planning has been associated with the success of community pharmacies.[6]

Like most humans, pharmacists prefer action to planning. It can be difficult for pharmacists to take time for systematic planning when the immediate course of action seems obvious.

Many pharmacists start important marketing initiatives with only a vague idea of what they want to do. They may say, "Let's provide pharmaceutical care to our patients. We can develop brochures to give to patients and charge $1 for each minute spent with the patient. Let's get started."

In businesses of all types, starting a new service with only a sketchy plan is not uncommon. However, such a plan often dooms the new service to failure, because it does not consider the many issues and problems involved in the success of a new idea.

Strategic marketing planning cannot be done successfully in one's head. It is important to compile a written marketing plan. Writing the plan helps focus ideas and ensures that important issues are not overlooked or

FIGURE 8-2 Steps in a strategic marketing plan. (Compiled from reference 7.)

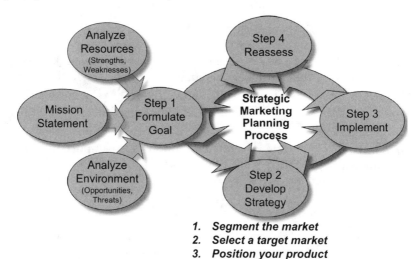

1. *Segment the market*
2. *Select a target market*
3. *Position your product*

ignored. A written plan prevents muddled thinking and makes it easier to share the plan with others.

SWOT ANALYSIS

The strategic marketing plan (Figure 8-2) is a step-by-step plan of action for solving marketing problems.[7] It starts with an analysis of the strengths (S) and weaknesses (W) of the marketing organization, followed by an evaluation of opportunities (O) and threats (T) in the market. Information from this *SWOT analysis* is used to develop and implement marketing goals and strategies. Then, the success of the plan is assessed to find flaws and failures. On the basis of this reassessment, marketing goals, strategies, and implementation plans are altered or discarded.

A marketing plan can be used any time there is a marketing problem. It can be executed when new services or changes in services are being considered, when a new competitor or major customer enters the market, or when any other event poses a problem for the marketer. The purpose of the marketing plan is to explicitly consider all major factors that might influence market success and then develop strategies to address them.

The S and W of SWOT analysis are an assessment of the organization's resources—its strengths and weaknesses within the market. To survive in a market, an organization has to capitalize on its strengths and overcome its weaknesses. The O and T are an environmental analysis of opportunities and threats in the market. Opportunities and threats often come from outside the organization and require an understanding of the world in which the organization operates.

SWOT analyses are conducted to support major marketing decisions. A SWOT analysis might be conducted when an organization is deciding about the feasibility of a new service (e.g., diabetes management). The purpose is to discover any distinct advantage for a pharmacy in the current environment, upon which a strategy can be built. SWOT analysis might also be used to discover any weaknesses that make a pharmacy vulnerable to competitors or prevent it from succeeding.

A clear understanding of the competition is an important part of SWOT analysis. Capabilities and the market environment are assessed by comparing the company with competitors. If location is considered a strength, it is a strength in comparison with competitors. Similarly, price is considered in relation to competitors' prices.

There are no cookbook methods for SWOT analysis. No two SWOT analyses are alike. Each depends on the market, competition, and characteristics of the marketing organization.

Capability (Strengths and Weaknesses) Assessment

A capability assessment attempts to clarify the current and potential capacity of an organization to compete in a market. It identifies strengths that give an organization an important advantage over competitors. These might include a well-known brand name, superior employees, strong company finances, or things the company is particularly good at doing. The capability assessment also identifies weaknesses that might hinder the company in the market. Weaknesses might include assets the company lacks or things the company does poorly in comparison with competitors.

One way to conduct a capability assessment is to take a sheet of paper and list your organization's strengths and weaknesses. Try to think of every characteristic of the business. Then use another sheet to list the strengths and weaknesses of competitors. If you do not have enough information to do this, you need to visit your competitors. Assessing the capability of competitors should suggest strengths and weaknesses to add to your own list.

Now use the lists for your organization and your competitors to complete the worksheet in Figure 8-3. Categorize the strengths and weaknesses as follows: people and skills (available personnel and their skills), money (availability of money to finance initiatives), systems (the quality

FIGURE 8-3 Worksheet for comparing your organization with competitors. For capabilities in which one organization has a competitive advantage over at least one other, put + in the column. For capabilities in which the organization has a disadvantage, put – in the column. For no advantage, put NA in the column.

Capability	Your Organization	Competitor A	Competitor B
People and skills			
Money			
Systems			
Facilities			
Market assets			

of the design and coordination of the organization), facilities (availability and condition of facilities), and market assets (the image and reputation of the organization in the eyes of consumers).

A simple capability assessment from a SWOT analysis of a diabetes management program at an independent pharmacy might look like Figure 8-4. The primary potential competitors for the independent's new diabetes management program are two nearby chain pharmacies, competitors A and B. Neither competitor currently has a diabetes management program. This SWOT analysis considers what might happen if either decided to offer such a program.

A quick glance shows that the independent's primary advantage over the competition is in personnel. The pharmacists at the independent are clinically trained and motivated to provide diabetes management services. If the owners of the independent pharmacy wished to strengthen the advantage, they could encourage one or more pharmacists to become certified diabetes educators. Two other advantages of the independent are its ability to quickly respond to changes and the reputation of the pharmacists in the community.

Only competitor B appears to be a threat to the independent pharmacy. Competitor A has few advantages and several disadvantages, compared with the independent and competitor B. Competitor B appears to have a clear advantage over the other two pharmacies in terms of money and facilities. Being part of a chain, it has greater financial resources than the independent. In addition, chain pharmacies can offer diabetes

FIGURE 8-4   Simplified capability assessment of an independent pharmacy's diabetes management program. Capabilities in which one organization has a competitive advantage over at least one other have + in the column. Capabilities in which the organization has a disadvantage have − in the column. NA means no organization has an advantage.

Capability	Your Organization	Competitor A	Competitor B
People and skills			
Clinically trained pharmacists	+	−	−
Clerkship training site	NA	NA	NA
Employee motivation to participate in program	+	−	+
Employees who are certified diabetes educators	NA	NA	NA
Money			
Availability of money to finance program	−	−	+
Willingness of management to wait for profitability	NA	NA	NA
Cash flow	−	−	+
Systems			
Ability of computer system to support program	NA	NA	NA
Ability to respond quickly to changes	+	−	−
Facilities			
Central location	NA	NA	NA
Ability to provide services in a large geographic area	−	+	+
Quality of patient counseling area	NA	NA	NA
Market assets			
Company's name is well recognized in the community	NA	NA	NA
Reputation of the pharmacists	+	−	−

management over a wide geographic area if the program is implemented throughout the chain. If it were able to develop a companywide program, the chain might better compete for diabetes management contracts with large managed care organizations.

Not all attributes of a company are equally important, and the importance of each attribute to the overall success of the strategic marketing plan should be considered. Perceptions of price are likely to be more important to the success of a disease management program than promotional displays are. One way to assess importance is to determine which attributes of the business are most difficult to copy. A company that has superior employees and managers has important advantages that are not easily duplicated.

Environmental (Opportunities and Threats) Analysis

Environmental analyses of opportunity and threat are conducted in concert with capability assessments. They are important in marketing plans because the environment has a significant effect on the relative capabilities of organizations and competitors. An influx of immigrants or the opening of a new factory in a community might give some firms an advantage over others.

An opportunity analysis identifies gaps between market demand and what is currently available. It also analyzes potential changes in the market that may enhance the prospects for services or products. An opportunity analysis might ask

- What needs are not being met in the current marketplace?
- How can our organization meet these needs better than competitors?
- How is the environment changing to the organization's advantage or disadvantage?

Opportunities can be found almost anywhere, if we keep our eyes open. One way of identifying opportunities is to continually scan the environment for new trends and changes. Opportunities can be found in discussions with customers, through reading magazines and newspapers and surfing the Internet, and by examining the trade literature.

Opportunities should be assessed for their desirability and their likelihood of success. Desirable opportunities are those most likely to generate a profit or make some contribution to the organization's mission. Likelihood of success is based on the capabilities of the organization, the capabilities of competitors, and the changing nature of the market.

A simple analysis of market opportunities for the diabetes management program described earlier might identify the following prospects for the program:

- More than 10% of the independent's current customers have diabetes.
- The current customers have sufficient income to pay for some services out of pocket if necessary.
- No other local pharmacies offer diabetes management at this time.
- Managed care payers have hinted that they may pay for diabetes services.

A threat analysis attempts to identify unfavorable factors that might injure the business. Like opportunities, threats are identified by scanning the environment for relevant trends and market changes. An analysis of threats should consider the seriousness of the threat as well as the likelihood of its occurring. A threat analysis might ask

- What potential problems might threaten the success of the organization's initiatives?
- What potential new competitors might arise? How might the organization's current competitors respond?
- What changes may be occurring in the environment to make our product or service obsolete?
- How might governmental policies, changing customer demographics, or a recession affect our organization's product or service?
- How might changes in customers' tastes affect demand?
- What major trends will significantly affect our organization and the market?

Threat analysis identifies situations that can be influenced by marketing actions and those that cannot. With situations that can be influenced, such as the entry of a major competitor into the area, problems can be minimized or even turned into opportunities if sufficient time is available. For instance, major competitors can sometimes thrive side by side if they offer a different mix of services and products. For situations that cannot be influenced, new ways of adapting must be found.

Porter[8] suggests that opportunities and threats can be identified by examining five characteristics of markets:

1. *The level of rivalry between competitors.* The more competitors there are fighting for customers, the less profitable and desirable a market is. When markets are saturated with competitors, opportunities are more limited than in growing markets. The only way to succeed in a competitive market is by taking customers away from competitors.
2. *The ease with which competitors can enter a market.* The harder it is for competitors to enter a market, the easier it is for those who remain to make a profit. It is harder to enter some markets than others. Barriers to entry into the pharmaceutical industry are very high. To develop and

manufacture pharmaceuticals in the United States, a company needs billions of dollars and vast resources. Entry into this market is restricted by government rules and laws, large start-up and operating costs, a need for highly trained and skilled personnel, and many other things. In comparison, the community pharmacy market is much easier to enter, although it still requires investment in facilities, technology, and personnel and is heavily regulated by local, state, and federal governments.

3. *The power of suppliers.* When suppliers of the inputs of a business are powerful, they can drive up the cost of inputs. For example, the high cost of pharmacist labor puts pressure on the profitability of pharmacy providers. Because of shortages in some parts of the country, qualified pharmacists have been able to demand higher salaries and greater job flexibility from employers. Similarly, a pharmaceutical company that has a unique and valued drug on the market can command high prices if no substitutes are available. Until a competing drug comes onto the market, drug companies can charge whatever the market will bear.

4. *The power of customers.* Large customers in a market can drive down prices and the profitability of businesses. With few other customers available, sellers are at a disadvantage. They are forced to negotiate better terms and prices with customers. Pharmacists have seen this situation occur when a few managed care organizations gain a significant share of the prescription drug market. Low dispensing fees for pharmacies are a consequence of the power of managed care. Likewise, the federal government is the largest purchaser of health care in the United States. Because of its power as a purchaser, the government can impose industrywide standards such as OBRA '90 (see Chapter 2) and force low prices on sellers.

5. *The availability of substitutes.* The greater the availability of substitutes for products and services, the more difficult it is for suppliers to charge higher prices and derive greater profits. A unique new drug on the market is often able to command high prices from purchasers unless substitutes can be found. When possible, managed care organizations attempt to use therapeutic alternatives or generic equivalents for more expensive brand name pharmaceuticals. The use of less expensive health care personnel is another example. Because physician services are so expensive, some health care providers use nurse practitioners and pharmacists in disease management and immunization programs. For expensive pharmacist positions, employers attempt to substitute more technology and technicians.

Any change in a market can present an opportunity or threat by affecting the level of rivalry, the ease of entry, the power of suppliers or customers, or the ability to substitute competing products or services. Other situations that can generate opportunities and threats are listed in Table 8-1.

TABLE 8-1   Situations That Can Generate Opportunities or Threats

Changes in the Business Climate
Recession
Expansion
New local businesses
Business closings

Changes in Consumer Preferences
Increasing use of herbal medicines
The move to self-treatment
Consumerism
Demand for convenience

Demographic Changes
Aging of America
Population shifts to the South
Population shifts to the suburbs
Immigration patterns

Legislative Changes
Local zoning
City government
State government
Federal government

Further analysis of the diabetes management program example might reveal the following threats:

■ Local nurse practitioners have just started to offer diabetes management at some physicians' offices.
■ The local hospital is considering the viability of a diabetes management program.
■ The state legislature has voted against collaborative practice programs and against officially designating pharmacists as health care professionals, thus hindering pharmacists' ability to receive compensation for services.

FORMULATING GOALS, OBJECTIVES, AND STRATEGIES

Once the SWOT analysis is completed and the information compiled, the pharmacist is able to begin setting marketing goals, objectives, and strategies. Goals and objectives are plans to achieve elements of success defined in the mission statement. Goals describe the general outcome of anticipated actions; an example is "To increase company profitability." Objectives quantify outcomes relating to goals; an example is "To increase return on assets by 10% by the end of the current fiscal year."

> *Marketing strategy must set forth a unique combination of price, product, place, and promotion—a combination that meets your customers' needs better than your competitors do.*

To be useful in decision-making, objectives must be realistic. They are meant to motivate people to achieve a goal that they can believe in. However, they are also meant to be challenging in order to stretch the abilities of those involved. Objectives must be specific and understandable so that people know what is expected. An objective like "work harder and faster" is not specific. A better objective might be to "increase prescription output by 10%." Finally, objectives must be measurable so that the organization knows when they have been accomplished.

Marketing strategy is the plan to achieve marketing goals and objectives. It describes what actions are to be taken in order to accomplish specific goals and objectives. Strategies for achieving a pharmacy's profitability goals and objectives might be to have sales on all major holidays, increase promotions of all high-margin merchandise, and discontinue the unprofitable greeting card department and use the space to expand the complementary medicine department.

The purpose of marketing strategy is to make customers prefer to do business with you rather than your competitors. Marketing strategy must set forth a unique combination of price, product, place, and promotion—a combination that meets your customers' needs better than your competitors do.

It is not sufficient that the quality of your product is higher. Many superior products fail on the market. Your product must also be priced, promoted, and located better than competitors' products.

Strategy boils down to three major steps: (1) segmenting your market, (2) targeting specific market segments, and (3) positioning your product in such a way that it will be purchased by your target market(s). Segmentation and targeting will be discussed in detail in Chapter 10. The following sections discuss positioning and a related topic, branding.

POSITIONING PHARMACEUTICAL SERVICES

Positioning strategy is the plan developed by marketers to communicate a desired, distinct image to customers. It is an effort to develop a marketing mix that provides a consistent and powerful image of your product or service. Promotion is a major component of any positioning strategy; however, price, place, and product also influence image. (See discussion of the marketing mix in Chapter 2.)

It is essential that your marketing mix be clear, distinct, and valued in the mind of your customer. If your customer does not perceive a clear benefit, then you have no advantage over your competitors. Businesses that do a poor job of differentiating themselves in the minds of customers become commodities.

A *commodity* is a product category that has no unique characteristics. When consumers cannot perceive any differences between products in a market, those products become a commodity. To most people, gasoline is a commodity. The gasoline at one gas station is considered as good as the gas at any other station, so quality is not an issue. As with most commodities, people tend to rely on price and location in selecting gas stations.

This example should cause some discomfort among pharmacists, since price and location are often cited as the primary reasons for selecting pharmacies. If price and location ever become the only reasons for selection, this will mean that pharmacies and pharmacists have not achieved a distinct perception of value in the minds of their patients— that they have become commodities. Pharmacists will have lost the marketing battle.

Successful positioning strategies use a marketing mix that is difficult to imitate. Although it may be easy for a competitor to imitate your patient education leaflets or brochures, it is difficult for a competitor to duplicate the interactions your pharmacists have with patients. The trust and friendships developed by pharmacists who are close to their customers cannot be copied. Individual pharmacists often provide a competitive advantage for their pharmacy.

The overarching goal of positioning is to give patients a reason to choose you over your competitors. You can accomplish this by identifying and highlighting your key advantages over your competition. By offering patients just one or two clear benefits, you can establish your competitive advantage.

> *Businesses that do a poor job of differentiating themselves in the minds of customers become commodities.*

BRANDS AND BRANDING

Branding is an important marketing activity associated with positioning. A *brand* is a name, term, sign, symbol, design, or some combination of these that is intended to identify the goods and services of one seller or group of sellers and to differentiate them from those of competitors.[7] *Branding* is the act of getting customers to attach some symbolic meaning to a brand.[7,9] People associate the word Tylenol with quality, value, and relief. Microsoft, Coke, and BMW are all associated with certain qualities in the minds of customers. Consumers who have positive perceptions of a brand are more likely to purchase or use that brand.

Walgreens, CVS, Rite Aid, Target, Kmart, Kroger, and Wal-Mart are common brands in pharmacy. Each is associated with a level of satisfaction, quality, and value in the mind of customers. Brands evoke responses that can range from hate to no opinion to fanatic loyalty. It is the marketer's goal to establish and enhance positive images for brands in the minds of customers.

The word *pharmacist* is a powerful brand in the minds of many customers. It may suggest images of trust, reliability, professionalism, and competence. For other people, however, it may bring to mind the image of pill counter or, almost as bad, it may evoke no image at all.

Individual pharmacists have their own brands: their names. Each pharmacist's name is associated with an image in the minds of those who interact with him or her. Think of a pharmacist you know who has a good reputation. What words come to mind when you think of that person? It is likely that your image of the pharmacist was the result of hard work on the part of that individual. Successful pharmacists take great care in developing and maintaining the image associated with their name.

Brand Awareness

Brand awareness is the strength of a brand's presence in a consumer's mind.[10] It is the extent to which consumers (1) recognize a brand when they see it (i.e., brand recognition) and (2) recall it when asked to consider the product category (i.e., brand recall).

Brand recognition comes from exposure such as advertising, previous experience, or recommendations from friends. Brand recognition means simply that when given a list of brands, consumers say they have heard of the brand. It is a weak measure of awareness.

Recognition is important because people are more positive toward familiar things.[10] For instance, most people would choose a food they have tasted over foods they have never tasted. If food looks different from food we have tried in the past, we resist trying it. It often takes marketing promotions or recommendations from friends and family members to get us to try a new food.

Brand recall means that consumers think of the brand when asked to list brands in a product category. It is a stronger measure of awareness than brand recognition. The percentage of people who answer "pharmacist" when asked, "Who is the drug expert among health care professionals?" is a measure of brand recall.

Brands that are quickly recalled are more likely to be considered in consumer choices.[10] In addition to recall of products and services, recall of individual people can be important. Mary Jones, the pharmacist, has a much better chance of being considered for a promotion if her name comes to mind when her bosses are discussing personnel matters. In other words, Mary cannot be considered if her name never comes up.

Brand Image

Brand image, also called brand meaning, refers to the dominant perception of a brand in consumers' minds.[11] It is the image that immediately comes to mind upon hearing a name such as Starbucks, McDonald's, Wal-Mart, or Microsoft. Brand image can be positive, neutral, or negative.

Brand image is determined by the types and quality of associations made in the minds of consumers. Associations can be made through sounds (e.g., musical jingles), visual images (e.g., logos), and words (e.g., slogans). Ideally, brand associations should be favorable to the brand and of sufficient strength and uniqueness to be recognized and recalled. Brand image comes from a variety of sources:

- *Customer experience.* Every contact with a branded object helps shape its image. For a pharmacy, image is shaped by the look of the parking lot, window signs, interior store appearance, and interactions with pharmacy personnel. For a pharmacist, image is shaped by general appearance, tone of voice, body language, and many other factors.
- *Promotional communications.* Television, radio, and newspaper advertising present images of pharmacies and pharmacists. Image comes from the portrayal of pharmacists and pharmaceuticals in promotional messages.
- *External information sources.* These include word-of-mouth recommendations from friends and family and publicity in the general press.

FIGURE 8-5 Brand equity model. (Compiled from reference 11.)

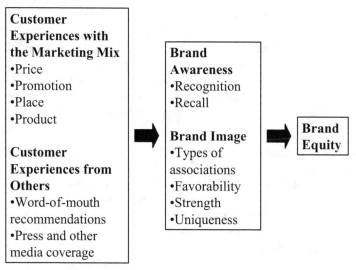

Sometimes promotional events can convey the wrong image of pharmacists. One grocery store chain decided to promote pharmacy services by giving away a 10- to 12-pound store-brand turkey with any two or more new or transferred prescriptions.[12] Such giveaways may be common practice for grocery stores, but associating pharmacists with turkeys may be inconsistent with the professional image pharmacists want to project.

Brand Equity

Branding provides value to a product. Consider branded laundry detergents. There is little actual difference between most laundry detergent brands, although their prices can vary considerably. The difference in price comes primarily from the brand image established through positioning. That difference in price is *brand equity*—the added value that a brand gives to a product or service.[10]

Brand equity is formed from a customer's awareness and perceived image of the brand (Figure 8-5).[11] Brand awareness and image come from personal experiences or through the communicated experiences of others. Each element of the marketing mix helps influence perceptions of the brand and brand equity. When a pharmacy gives away professional services to patients or promotes low prescription drug prices, that affects the image of professional services. To protect the equity of the brand, pharmacists must carefully consider how marketing actions affect brand perceptions.

Although some critics might say that branding does nothing but add extra cost for the consumer, the consumer can benefit from branding. Branding can simplify the consumer's search for a product. The consumer simply looks for the trusted brand and makes the purchase. A good brand image can also reduce the buyer's perceived risk of making a bad decision. For instance, patients with serious health conditions tend to seek out physicians with the best reputation. Although other physicians may be equally good, the physician with the best reputation is the one most in demand. The greater the risk, the more important branding becomes in making a choice.

Marketers measure brand equity in two ways. The first is to assess consumer perceptions of the brand through studies of reputation or image. A strong reputation can help differentiate a seller's products and services from those of competitors. The second way to measure brand equity is to calculate the financial value added to a product as a result of increased sales and profits. Strong brands permit sellers to charge higher prices and derive greater profits.

Patients' image of pharmacies and individual pharmacists has a substantial influence on their loyalty, buying habits, and willingness to participate in therapy. Pharmacists and pharmacies that are able to project and maintain a positive brand image in the minds of customers are more likely to achieve success both professionally and financially.

Sometimes a brand must be changed, such as when the 400-store Peoples Drug chain was purchased by the CVS pharmacy chain.[13] CVS had to decide whether to keep the Peoples Drug name on the new stores and retain Peoples brand equity or to change all of the new stores to the CVS brand. CVS used a brand image study to better understand the market served by Peoples and determine if a name change would be successful. Initially, the change appeared risky, since Peoples was a strongly established household name in the markets it served. However, the study identified a tone and approach to advertising and brand positioning that CVS could use to emphasize both innovation and continuity. With the slogan "Same thing only better," CVS was able to implement the name change.

Changing Your Brand's Image

If customers' current image of your brand is not the image you desire, you need to reposition the brand in a way that closes the gap between the actual and the desired image.

Aaker[10] describes a "trap" that occurs when marketers are not willing or able to do what is necessary to change the current brand image to the desired image. An example can be seen in pharmacy: Many pharmacists, although unhappy with their professional image, are unwilling to expend the effort necessary to change people's minds. Rather than change the current image of the profession, they become frustrated and accept things as they are. They adapt to the perceptions of others rather than clearly defining what they stand for. They are still trying to decide whether they want to move

> *Pharmacists must improve their brand image in the minds of both their patients and their employers.*

beyond their current image and shape a new one. Pharmacists can use the checklist on page 174 to assess how effectively they are promoting their brand image.

One reason for the gap between the desired and current image of pharmacists is that many pharmacists do not exert much control in their practice environment. Leventhal[14] argues that entities with brands need to control the core assets associated with the brand. Coke and Pepsi own the recipe, brand name, and image associated with their products. The Walt Disney Company owns its core assets. But, in many cases, the profession of pharmacy does not own its core assets. The product and the promotion of pharmacist image are controlled primarily by large corporations that may not appreciate the pharmacist brand. Pharmacists need to promote the desired image of the profession to customers both inside and outside pharmacy organizations. Pharmacists must improve their brand image in the minds of both their patients and their employers.

IMPLEMENTING THE MARKETING PLAN

Even the best-conceived marketing plans can fail if they are poorly implemented.[10,15] Successful implementation of marketing plans can be hindered in several ways. Sometimes poor implementation is just a failure to follow the plan. This can occur when not all people in the organization understand the plan and their roles. In other cases, implementation may suffer if people lose sight of the mission. In still other situations, structural limitations of the business can limit the success of some ideas. Bonoma[15] has described the following problems associated with implementation.

Insufficient commitment from management. When XYZ pharmacy decides to offer disease management services as part of its strategy, upper management of XYZ can hurt the implementation if it is not sufficiently committed to the idea. Lack of commitment may cause management to do things that make success difficult. Management may cut funding or staff. Consider the following example of a disease management program that management did not permit to succeed.

Tomasin's Pharmacy (name changed) was beginning to achieve some success in disease management services. The pharmacy was building national recognition for its innovative services in smoking cessation and diabetes management. However, pharmacy management was uncomfortable with the idea of clinical services and decided to reduce efforts in this area. A decision was made to emphasize basic dispensing services, with which managers were more familiar, over clinical services. Pharmacists were pressured to cut back their disease management efforts. The pharmacy management thought that emphasizing dispensing would have greater impact on the sale of nonprescription merchandise, the most profitable part of the business. Management believed that clinical services would be too risky and require too many resources.

Here, the strategy to provide innovative services failed, but not because it was a bad idea. It failed because pharmacy management was not sufficiently committed. The merchandising plans of the company made it much easier for pharmacy management to stick with familiar dispensing services rather than clinical services. Management was more interested in using the pharmacy department to enhance store traffic than in meeting customers' health care needs.

Lack of staff commitment or expertise. Implementation can also fail because of insufficient commitment or expertise at the staff level. The best plan in the world will fail if people are unwilling or unable to follow it. A marketing plan that does not take into account the strengths and limitations of employees and managers in a company is likely to fail. For example, the implementation of medication therapy management services requires pharmacists who are competent, flexible, and enthusiastic about challenges. Not all pharmacists fit this description. Some are just not interested in stepping outside their traditional dispensing roles. Others may be uncomfortable with new tasks, or interested but not trained in providing higher levels of care. If such human limitations are not addressed, the marketing plan can fail.

Insufficient or bad information. Many marketing decisions are made with bad or insufficient information. Decisions are based on faulty assumptions about the business and the market. If managers assume that consumers care about only price and convenience, they will ignore the potential for patient care services. If managers lack information about competitors, customers, and the market, they will rely on past experience or assumptions that may not be relevant or appropriate to current conditions.

Structural contradictions. Marketing strategy often dictates a course of action that is inconsistent with the structural characteristics of the organization. Strategy may recommend that employees take greater responsibility in handling customers, while employee personnel policies inhibit or even punish employees who do so. Marketing strategies must be developed with explicit consideration of the structural characteristics of the organization. Successful implementation of marketing plans may require changes in structural aspects of the business, such as operating procedures and redesign of workflow and facilities.

Overextension. In most organizations, there are too many marketing tasks to accomplish with current resources and personnel. As a result, company leaders often try to do too many things and are unable to do any of them well. A pharmacy may wish to provide outstanding dispensing services, on-demand immunizations and clinical services, community outreach, and patient callbacks. Trying to do all of these things may result in failure of all of them. Successful implementation requires that choices be made.

REASSESSING

A feedback and control system should be put in place to evaluate the success of programs and identify ways in which they can be improved. Such a system could consist of a scheduled review of marketing programs and an action plan to address problems.

At the beginning of any program, a decision needs to be made about how to determine whether it is successful. This requires that measures of success or failure be collected. Measures of successful pharmacy services might consist of the total number of patients who use the service, revenue collected from the service, and patient satisfaction. The key is to identify the minimum number of easy-to-collect measures that can validly determine the success of the program.

When it is time to evaluate a program, a decision can be made to continue the program without changes, cancel the program, or make changes. Changes can include expansion of programs, contraction of programs, or adjustments designed to improve programs. In an ideal situation, a continuous quality improvement method should be used (see Chapter 4). Continuous quality improvement consists of applying the best methods from the literature to the pharmacy's own practice, using statistical quality improvement techniques to measure the results, and then using what was learned to make improvements. Pharmacists may choose instead to rely on their own personal judgment when reassessing efforts. A pharmacist who maintains close contact with the operations and patients of a pharmacy probably has a good idea of which strategies work and which do not, without the need for extensive statistical analyses.

Branding Checklist for Pharmacists

How do you differ from the average pharmacist? What makes your pharmacy different from other pharmacies in the community? To attract patients for you to serve, you must persuade them to choose you over your competitors. Your patients must believe you give them something that your competitors do not. This requires you to develop a clear, positive, strong brand that people recognize.

Pharmacists should continually ask themselves what image they present and assess how patients see them. This checklist can be used to evaluate the effectiveness of your branding strategy.

❑ We have a clearly defined brand image that we want to communicate to our patients. (If you do not have a clear image, how can your patients have one?)

❑ Everyone on our team shares a similar vision of what our brand should be. (A shared vision is important because your brand is determined in large part by the actions of each individual on your team.)

❑ Everyone on our team can articulate a shared vision of what our brand should be. (Being able to articulate your image requires a greater level of comprehension and commitment to a brand than does simply sharing a vision. Team members who can verbalize what you stand for can better promote your brand to patients.)

❑ We can list the unique elements of value that we provide to our patients. (If you do not identify the unique value you provide, it will be impossible to convince patients of how your brand differs from others.)

❑ We can list the unique elements of value offered by our competitors. (You need to know the value your competitors provide in order to identify why you are better.)

❑ We tailor our promotional communications to support and enhance our brand. (Advertising, public relations, personal selling, and all other forms of promotional communications should provide a consistent image of your brand. Inconsistencies in communications can result in a garbled image in the minds of patients.)

❑ All elements of our business (e.g., pharmacy, front end, promotions, Web site) communicate the same brand image. (Every contact with your patients communicates an image to them. Everything they see, hear, smell, touch, and taste says something about your brand. Make certain that the message is what you want to convey.)

❑ Our patients know pharmacy personnel and ask for us by our names. (The brands of frontline personnel reinforce the brands of pharmacies. Patients who know and ask for their pharmacists will have greater brand loyalty.)

❑ We continually solicit patient perceptions about our brand. (Brand image is constantly evolving and renewing with each patient contact. It is essential that brand meaning, awareness, and recall be constantly assessed.)

SUMMARY

The ability to develop a strategic marketing plan is an important skill for pharmacists who wish to market their services. The steps to strategic marketing planning have been presented in a way that permits any pharmacist to write and implement a plan.

Marketing is not an event, but a process.... It has a beginning, a middle, but never an end, for it is a process. You improve it, perfect it, change it, even pause it. But you never stop it completely.

Jay Conrad Levinson, advocate of "guerrilla marketing"

References

1. American Pharmacists Association. APhA mission, vision, values, and strategic goals. Available at: www.aphanet.org. Accessed March 7, 2007.
2. Rite Aid Corporation. Rite Aid's core values and mission. Available at: www.riteaid.com. Accessed March 7, 2007.
3. Virginia Commonwealth University School of Pharmacy Mission Statement. Available at: www.pharmacy.vcu.edu/annualreport/index.html. Accessed March 7, 2007.
4. Franzak FJ. The use of marketing strategy by pharmacists. *Health Mark Q.* 1992;9:133–41.
5. Harrison DL, Ortmeier BG. Strategic planning in the community pharmacy. *J Am Pharm Assoc.* 1996;NS36:583–8.
6. McGee JE, Love LG, Festervand TA. Competitive advantage and the independent retail pharmacy: the role of distinctive competencies. *J Pharm Mark Manage.* 2000;13:31–46.
7. Kotler P. *Marketing Management: Analysis, Planning, and Control.* 4th ed. Englewood Cliffs, NJ: Prentice Hall; 1980.
8. Porter ME. *Competitive Strategy: Techniques for Analyzing Industries and Competition.* New York: The Free Press; 1980.
9. Berry LL. Cultivating service brand equity. *J Acad Mark Sci.* 2000;28: 128–37.
10. Aaker DA. *Building Strong Brands.* New York: The Free Press; 1996.
11. Keller KL. Conceptualizing, measuring, and managing customer-based brand equity. *J Mark.* 1993;57:1–22.
12. Slezak M. Winn-Dixie ties turkey sales to pharmacy. *Supermarket News.* 1994;44(47):35.
13. Kolligan MK. What's in a name? The conversion of Peoples Drug to CVS. *J Advert Res.* 1998;38(6):46.
14. Leventhal RC. Branding strategy. *Bus Horiz.* September–October 1996;35: 17–23.
15. Bonoma TV. Making your marketing strategy work. *Harv Bus Rev.* March–April 1984;62:69–78.

Additional Readings

Doucette WR, McDonough RP, Klepser D, et al. Comprehensive medication therapy management: identifying and resolving drug-related issues in a community pharmacy. *Clin Ther.* 2005;27(7)1104–11.

Garrett DG, Martin LA. The Asheville Project: participants' perceptions of factors contributing to the success of a patient self-management diabetes program. *J Am Pharm Assoc.* 2003;43:185–90.

McDonough RP, Rovers JP, Currie JD, et al. Obstacles to the implementation of pharmaceutical care in the community setting. *J Am Pharm Assoc.* 1998; 38:87–95.

Medication therapy management services: a critical review. *J Am Pharm Assoc.* 2005;45:580–7.

Exercises and Questions

1. Write a mission statement for a pharmacy where you would want to work.
2. How do pharmaceutical care or other clinical services fit into the overall business plan of your current or previous pharmacy employer?
3. What is the purpose of a SWOT analysis? When should it be conducted? Why is knowledge of the competition important in a SWOT analysis?
4. Porter suggests five characteristics of markets that affect their desirability. Use them to describe the desirability of a pharmacy service or product (of your choice) in the market. For instance, what substitutes are available to customers?
5. What are the differences between goals, objectives, and strategies? What are the characteristics of a good objective?
6. Compare and contrast brand image, brand recall, brand equity, and brand awareness, using your name as the "brand."
7. Describe common pharmacy practices that you believe enhance or hurt the image of pharmacists as health care professionals.
8. Name the first three community pharmacy brands that come to your mind. What images do you associate with these brands? In what ways are the brand images similar? Different?

Activity

Conduct a SWOT analysis of the market for a pharmacy program or service.

MARKETING STRATEGIES

Independent pharmacists use a variety of marketing strategies to compete with large pharmacy chains. A *Wall Street Journal* article[1] described some strategies that one independent, which is surrounded by chain stores, has used to survive and even thrive:

Personalized service: Employees greet patrons by name at the entrance, arrange for patients' prescriptions to be picked up after hours—and even program the remote control that an elderly customer has just purchased for his VCR.

Imaginative merchandising, facilities, and products not offered by chains.

Targeting specific customer groups such as senior citizens.

Offering a broad range of services such as photocopying, filling same-day special orders, and accepting IOUs from cash-strapped patients.

Competitive pricing of merchandise through aggressive buying and taking advantage of manufacturer discounts.

Neutralizing the chains' price advantage by offering competitive prices on the top 200 prescription drugs, even if it means selling the drugs at cost.

Advertising in local promotional circulars and offering $5-off prescription coupons.

Hiring additional pharmacists so more time can be spent with patients and professional services such as blood pressure and diabetes screenings can be offered.

Numerous business articles and books—indeed, whole sections of bookstores—are devoted to strategies for marketing products and services. This chapter discusses some strategies that can be applied to pharmacy practice.

PORTER'S GENERIC MARKETING STRATEGIES

Porter[2] argues that all generic business strategies are determined by the business's source of competitive advantage (low cost or differentiation) and scope of targeted markets (broad or narrow) (Figure 9-1). In other words, businesses compete on the basis of cost, differentiation, and focus, and all business strategies are some variation on these three approaches.

FIGURE 9-1 Porter's generic marketing strategies. (Compiled from reference 2.)

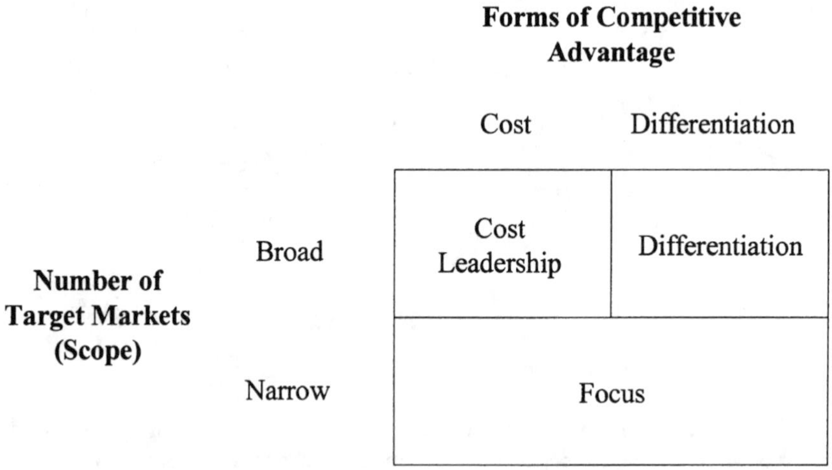

Forms of Competitive Advantage

		Cost	Differentiation
Number of Target Markets (Scope)	Broad	Cost Leadership	Differentiation
	Narrow	Focus	

Businesses gain advantage in markets by being cheaper than competitors, being different in some recognizable and valuable way, or serving narrow market segments.

Cost Strategies

Cost-based strategies identify and exploit opportunities to reduce costs below competitors' costs, primarily by being more efficient, and to drive down prices. Efficiency can be increased by designing workplace environments that simplify and facilitate work, using systems that reduce wasted effort, targeting customers who are more profitable to the firm, motivating employees to work harder and smarter, and so on.

Within their market, cost leaders compete by undercutting the prices of competitors. Winning customer volume away from competitors makes up for lower profit margins and enables the business to remain profitable. Profits are then used to develop new ways of doing business that further reduce cost.

Wal-Mart department stores are famous for their low-cost business strategy. Wal-Mart uses its tremendous purchasing power and efficient supply chain to provide products at a lower average price than most competitors. When unable or unwilling to compete with Wal-Mart in terms of price, competitors use other strategies.[3,4]

Differentiation Strategies

Price becomes less important when businesses compete by offering a product or service package that is of higher quality, performs better, or is uniquely desirable. Businesses that differentiate themselves from competitors do so by offering a distinctive mix of products and services that are highlighted by effective advertising and promotion.

Differentiation strategies emphasize value more than price competition. Customers buy differentiated products and services because they perceive that they are getting more for their money. A desire for the lowest price is replaced by a desire for the highest value. Pharmacies often try to differentiate themselves from competitors by providing greater levels of service. This might mean faster, friendlier, more varied, or more convenient service.

Customers buy differentiated products and services because they perceive that they are getting more for their money.

Medicine Shoppe, an international chain of franchise pharmacies, uses a differentiation strategy.[5] In 2006, the chain had

900 Medicine Shoppe and Medicap pharmacies in the United States and 400 in seven other countries.[6] Medicine Shoppes differentiate themselves from the average pharmacy by being small (averaging 600 square feet) and oriented more toward health care than toward general merchandise. The pharmacy front end does not contain the large array of food, greeting cards, and other nonhealth products found in a typical pharmacy. In fact, 96% of the chain's sales come from the pharmacy. The limited front-end merchandise is health related. Since most Medicine Shoppe pharmacists are franchise owners, customers deal directly with the owner, not an employee.

Focus Strategies

While differentiation strategies target large customer populations, focus strategies identify narrow market segments (or niches) that have been ignored, overlooked, or taken for granted by competitors. Many independent pharmacies successfully compete with large chains by giving greater attention to the local community. Focusing on narrow geographic niches, independent pharmacists are often active in local organizations and more familiar with neighborhood needs and interests than are employees of large chains. Their closeness to the community can generate goodwill that gives them a competitive advantage over larger firms.

This type of strategy focuses on the needs of a profitable few. Rather than compete for all customers in a market, firms compete for a limited number of profitable customers whom the firms can serve better than their competitors can. Pharmacists have attempted to serve the following niches: diabetes, asthma, cholesterol, lab services, reproductive health, vaccines, hospice, AIDS, veterinary services, smoking cessation, hypertension, complementary medicines, anticoagulation services, and postal delivery.

Choosing an Approach

The appropriate strategy to choose—low cost, differentiation, or focus—depends on the market situation and a firm's capabilities. A single independent pharmacy may find that focus strategies are the only way to compete with large pharmacy chains, because of the vast resources available to chains. A small pharmacy chain may find it too difficult to be cost competitive with a larger competitor that has significant cost advantages in distribution and operations. Instead, the chain might find a unique way to differentiate itself. A large pharmacy chain that is a market leader might develop economies of scale to reduce costs.

No one strategy is necessarily better than any other. The only measure of which one is best for an individual firm is its success in the market. Porter cautions, however, that it is important to choose only one of these

FIGURE 9-2   Sales and profits within a product's life cycle. (Compiled from reference 7.)

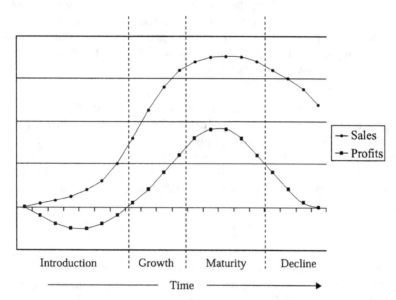

strategies. A business needs to choose a single strategy and become proficient at it. Use of a single strategy also helps present a consistent image of the business to consumers.

PRODUCT LIFE-CYCLE STRATEGIES

The idea of product life cycles is that, like plants and animals, products have a life. Each product life cycle has four stages: introduction, growth, maturity, and decline.[7] Sales volume and profitability vary over time as products progress through each stage (Figure 9-2). By identifying a product's life-cycle stage, a marketer can develop strategies with increased chances for success.

The product life-cycle concept permits a business to understand sales of a single product within a market. Life-cycle strategies are most commonly used for products that are exceptional, meet an unrealized need, and are unknown to the general market.

Introduction

New products or brands in the introduction stage are unique and face no immediate, direct competition. The goal of marketing is to introduce the product to consumers and induce them to try it. Since the product is new, sales growth is slow initially and profits are negative. The amount of money spent on promoting the product exceeds the revenue from sales. Promotional dollars are spent to educate consumers about the product's existence. Sales promotions, coupons, and price discounts attempt to persuade consumers to try the product. Money put into the product at this stage is an investment that the business hopes will pay off in later stages of the life cycle.

In community pharmacy practice, most clinical services are still in the introduction stage. These services fulfill a latent need, but they are often not profitable because they are not widely known or accepted. Significant money and effort still need to be expended before these services can move into the growth stage. Unless sufficient effort is spent promoting clinical services in community pharmacy, they risk dying a premature death.

Growth

In the growth stage, demand for the product starts to rise. Sales accelerate rapidly, climbing initially at an increasing pace and then at a decreasing rate toward the end of the growth stage. Since there are few competitors in the market at the beginning of the growth stage, high prices can be charged, and profits start to move into positive territory.

As the product moves through the growth stage, competitors start to enter the market to gain a share of the profits. This puts pressure on prices and profits. Early entrants into the market must either lower prices in response or offer innovations that justify higher prices. The first, innovative product on the market typically has an advantage over later market entrants, because significant experience and brand awareness can be gained in the introduction stage. This experience can be used to stay one step ahead of competitors.

Maturity

In the maturity stage, sales reach their peak and start to decline. Profits start to erode. This stage is typically the longest one; for some products it can last decades. Although profits start to decline in the maturity stage, they can still be sufficient. In this stage, the goal of marketers is to defend their share of the market from competitors. This can be done by constantly refining the marketing mix.

Dispensing services have been in the maturity stage for many years. They are unchanged in many respects from 50 years ago. Most competition in dispensing has been through minor improvements designed to attract different market segments, improve quality, and drive down prices. Innovations such as drive-through windows, Internet services, and telephone refill services have permitted pharmacies to prolong the maturity phase of dispensing services.

Decline

During this stage, sales and profits decrease until the product is withdrawn from the market. Like any living organism, a product reaches a stage where it can no longer survive. Consumer tastes may change, or a new competitor may dry up demand in the market. Whatever the reason, products eventually decline and disappear from the market. Manual typewriters and the slide rule eventually disappeared from the market, and this will happen to many services and products provided by pharmacists.

Alternative Life Cycles

The classic S shape of the original life-cycle model does not always accurately describe a product's life pattern. In some cases a product's life cycle is a series of S shapes (Figure 9-3). This pattern is common with prescription drugs.[8,9] Drugs follow this cycle–recycle pattern when a product is first introduced as a prescription medication and then reintroduced at a later date with new selling features, such as a new disease indication, modified dosage forms, or nonprescription status.

FIGURE 9-3   Cycle–recycle product life-cycle model.

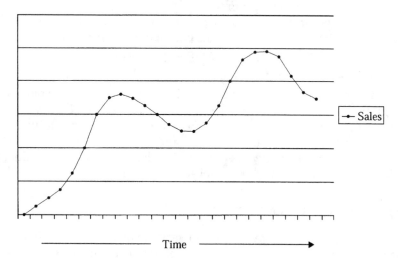

The ulcer drug Zantac (ranitidine; Pfizer) can be used to illustrate the cycle–recycle pattern. The H_2-receptor antagonist was approved by the Food and Drug Administration in 1983 for the treatment of peptic ulcer. The market for Zantac expanded over the years as the following events occurred:[10]

- The manufacturer's target market changed from gastroenterologists to primary care physicians.
- An intravenous dosage form was introduced in 1984.
- Zantac was approved for short-term treatment of gastric ulcer in 1985.
- Zantac was approved for maintenance therapy of duodenal ulcer and treatment of gastroesophageal reflux disease in 1986.
- Direct-to-consumer advertising started in the late 1980s.
- Zantac was approved for long-term use to prevent duodenal ulcer in 1989.
- Effervescent and gel dosage forms of Zantac were introduced in 1994.
- Nonprescription Zantac was launched in 1996.

Throughout this period, Zantac had to respond to competition from other H_2 antagonists, proton pump inhibitors, and generic ranitidine. Through excellent strategic marketing decisions, the marketers of Zantac have been able to extend its life to the present day.

Lessons from the Product Life Cycle

Understanding product life cycles provides perspective for pharmacists who implement new programs. Any new idea, such as pharmaceutical care, takes time and effort to bear fruit. During the introduction stage, time, effort, and patience on the part of the pharmacist are required. Pharmacists should not expect immediate payoff.

If an idea is successful enough to move into the desirable growth stage, a lot of work needs to be done to keep it there. As business explodes in the growth stage, demand may look as if it will never end. However, as competitors move into growing markets, it is more difficult to increase and sustain sales and profits. As an idea moves into the maturity stage, it takes constant marketing to keep it thriving. Finally, when the product is no longer profitable, it must be removed from the market.

PORTFOLIO STRATEGIES

A portfolio is all the products and services offered by a business. A portfolio strategy helps define the mix of products and services that a

FIGURE 9-4   Portfolio matrix. (Compiled from reference 11.)

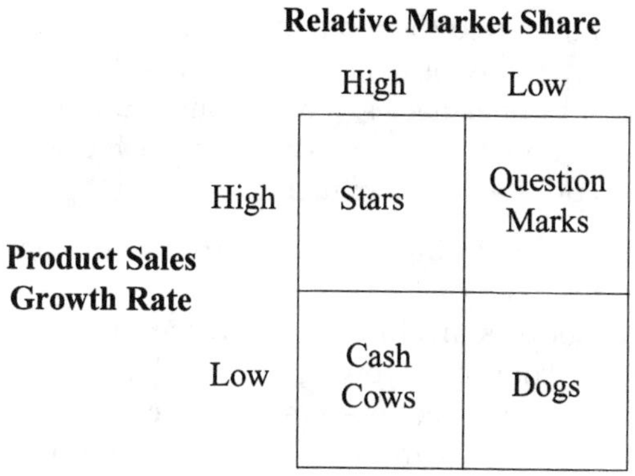

Relative Market Share

	High	Low
High	Stars	Question Marks
Low	Cash Cows	Dogs

Product Sales Growth Rate

business offers. The Boston Consulting Group developed a way to display products in a portfolio matrix that helps drive marketing actions (Figure 9-4).[11] Products within the matrix are classified by market share and sales growth rate. Use of the matrix helps determine whether a product should receive greater investments, have its cash flow harvested for other parts of the business, or be dropped from the portfolio. Figure 9-5 shows the portfolio of a hypothetical pharmacy chain.

FIGURE 9-5   Portfolio matrix for a hypothetical chain pharmacy. OTC = over-the-counter (nonprescription).

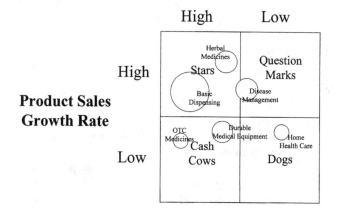

Relative Market Share

Within the matrix, "cash cows" are products with a high market share in a low-growth market. Cash cows generate excess cash for a business, which can then be allocated to help develop and promote other products. The strategy with cash cows is to milk them for cash and provide minimal input of resources. In pharmacies, many front-end merchandise sections (e.g., greeting cards and photo processing) are cash cows that are used to finance other, less profitable departments.

"Stars" are products in high-growth, large-share markets. Although growing, stars offer potential for even greater future growth. Because of their potential, resources are invested in these products. As their market matures, they become cash cows. Internet pharmacy services in some businesses might be classified as stars. They are a fast-growing market, and their potential justifies the money spent on promoting them and building their infrastructure.

"Question marks" are products with weak market positions in high growth rate markets. Improving on their weak market position will require significant effort. If the potential benefit of a question mark product is not worth the cost, the business may decide to put its efforts elsewhere.

"Dogs" are products with a low market share in low-growth markets. They provide little value to the business and can be a drain on resources. Dogs are candidates for withdrawal from the market.

Most community pharmacies offer a variety of prescription and non-prescription merchandise and services. Combining the product life-cycle approach with the portfolio strategy can help in evaluating each product and service for its current and potential contribution to the whole portfolio.

To serve the needs of different market segments, pharmacists need to provide a flexible portfolio of services. Pharmacies have developed different product and service offerings to serve various customer market segments; often information about a pharmacy's portfolio can be found on its Web site. Pharmacies' strategies for competing in the market can be identified by comparing their portfolios.

To assess and fine tune a pharmacy service portfolio, pharmacists need to follow several steps.

1. Identify your primary target markets, such as patients with certain disease states, patients of particular physicians, certain age groups, or managed care customers.
2. Inventory your current service offerings. Most pharmacies provide basic dispensing services that are supported by front-end merchandise purchases. Other potential services might be counseling, disease

management, screening for conditions such as osteoporosis, vaccinations, durable goods fittings, home health care, and nursing home services.
3. Identify which of your current services are viable in your target markets. The goal is to offer different levels of services depending on the target market. For instance, managed care companies may be open to proposals for certain disease management or vaccination programs that complement basic dispensing services. Seniors may be willing to pay for extensive counseling about their prescriptions.
4. Identify which services you need to add or subtract to round out your service portfolio. Selection depends on the value of each service to your various target markets and the cost of providing the service. Services can be assessed for their importance to customers, customer willingness to pay, and a service's overall contribution to the service portfolio. The goal is to match the right services to the needs of target segments at the lowest costs.

An additional consideration in evaluating a product or service is how it might help balance the portfolio. Although some products do not generate much cash or have high growth potential, they can add balance to the overall portfolio. A cholesterol screening program might not generate much immediate revenue for the pharmacy or have much potential for doing so in the future. However, it can benefit the product and service portfolio of the pharmacy by complementing the other disease management offerings, generating store traffic, and enhancing the image of the pharmacy in the community.

CONVENIENCE STRATEGIES

A major way that pharmacies differentiate themselves is through convenience strategies. Most community pharmacies have made convenience an important part of their overall marketing strategy. This makes sense, because research has consistently found location and convenience to be important factors in consumer patronage of pharmacies.[12] In fact, pharmacy uses convenience to differentiate itself from other professions, referring to the pharmacist as the "most accessible health care professional."

Convenience generally refers to speed and ease of shopping. This includes the ability to shop at one location, availability of store directories, clearly marked merchandise and prices, a good store layout, easy traffic flow in the aisles, minimal out-of-stock merchandise, no waiting in lines, and expanded operating hours.[13]

But convenience means different things to different people. For parents with small children, it might mean having prescriptions filled without getting out of the car. For a housebound disabled person, it might mean being able to shop from home. For a young, healthy shopper, it might mean easy parking and one-stop shopping for clothing, groceries, household goods, and drugs.

The push for customer convenience has been responsible for many changes in the practice of pharmacy. Convenience is the reason pharmacies are located in supermarkets, shopping malls, and mass merchandisers (e.g., Target, Kmart, and Wal-Mart). It is the reason for drive-through, mail order, and Internet pharmacies.

The Downside of Convenience Strategies

One problem with convenience strategies is that the demand for greater convenience never ends.[13] Each time a pharmacy offers a convenience innovation, consumers quickly become accustomed to it and expect further improvement. Moreover, the advantage of a convenience improvement fades when competitors copy it. Also, innovations of nonpharmacy businesses raise consumer expectations of convenience. When consumers see that a bank transaction worth thousands of dollars can be completed in 30 seconds, they begin to wonder why a prescription can't be filled in the same amount of time.

Pharmacy services that are now considered convenient will be regarded as slow in the future. Consider 24-hour photo processing. Consumers used to wait days or weeks to have photographs developed and returned to them. Pharmacies started offering 24-hour photo processing, but some consumers soon found this too slow. Now, 24-hour processing competes with 1-hour processing and processing while the customer waits. Consumers who want even greater convenience can use a digital camera and see their photos immediately after they take them.

Competing on the basis of convenience takes tremendous commitment and continuous hard work to stay ahead of competitors. Also, convenience strategies can be expensive. Keeping customer checkout lines short may require pharmacy managers to increase staffing. Hiring pharmacists to work extended hours can necessitate higher salaries. Pharmacies may find the cost of many convenience strategies to be prohibitive.

Finally, reliance on convenience strategies can have a negative impact on the professional image of pharmacists. High-volume, low-service pharmacies can hurt the public's perception of the professional effort that goes into filling each prescription. Drive-through pharmacies may lead consumers to associate pharmacists more with fast food restaurants than with health care services. Little research is available regarding the impact of convenience strategies on pharmacist image—but think about how consumers would view physicians if they provided consultations at a drive-through window.

Types of Convenience

Seiders et al.[13] identify four aspects of convenience to consider in developing marketing strategies. Each requires different actions on the part of marketers. It is important that pharmacists define the aspect of convenience they want to promote. The four are

1. *Access convenience:* Easy to reach,
2. *Search convenience:* Easy to identify and select,
3. *Possession convenience:* Easy to obtain, and
4. *Transaction convenience:* Easy to purchase and return.

Access Convenience

Access convenience refers to the speed and ease with which customers can reach the pharmacist in person, by telephone, over the Internet, or by mail. It is affected by factors such as the location of the pharmacy, ease of parking, hours of business, convenience to other businesses of interest, telephone systems, and Internet access.[13]

Location is one of the top attributes used in choosing pharmacy services. It can mean the difference between succeeding and going out of business. The importance of location has led to an area of marketing expertise called location analysis, which addresses factors that determine the success or failure of business locations. One common strategy is to locate pharmacies in standalone settings next to busy intersections. Placing stores on busy street corners allows customers to stop at pharmacies on their way to other destinations. Keeping pharmacies separate from other businesses allows drive-through lanes and windows to be installed. Standalone locations also separate pharmacies from competitors such as grocery stores and mass merchandisers. Walgreens uses this location strategy.[13]

An alternative convenience strategy is to locate pharmacies close to other businesses. Locating a pharmacy next to businesses with a complementary mix of products and services allows customers one-stop shopping. Strip mall pharmacies may locate near businesses whose customers might stop by the pharmacy before or after a visit. Clinic pharmacies may be located in or next to physicians' offices and hospitals. A variation of locating pharmacies next to businesses is to locate them inside businesses. Grocery stores and mass merchandisers have adopted this strategy.

In addition to location, access convenience considers the ease with which pharmacy customers can get into a pharmacy from the parking lot and back out again. If consumers must wait for an open parking space or park far away from the pharmacy, they may decide that a visit to the pharmacy is not worth the effort.

Search Convenience

Search convenience refers to how easily customers can identify and select the products and services they want to buy. When the search for pharmacy products is difficult, customers are likely to become frustrated and leave the pharmacy empty-handed and unsatisfied. Low search convenience can also increase consumer anxiety.

Search convenience can be enhanced by clear and available signs at the spots where people need them, a sensible pharmacy layout and design, knowledgeable and helpful personnel who can assist consumers, and customized interactive technology.[13] The more the pharmacy does to facilitate the search process, the better shopping experience the customer has.

Pharmacists can make the search easier by keeping an eye out for customers who need help and providing assistance. This can mean more than just pointing in a general direction or stating an aisle number. The regional grocery store chain Ukrop's trains all employees, including pharmacists, to accompany the customer to the location of the item of interest and find the product on the shelf.

For people who like to help themselves, interactive kiosks can provide information about pharmacy products or health conditions. Electronic gift registries are common for weddings, showers, and graduation. Such interactive registries may become more common in pharmacies.

Possession Convenience

Possession convenience refers to the ease of acquiring a product or service—whether products are in stock and the process involved in receiving the product. Most national and regional pharmacy chains enhance possession convenience by permitting patients to have their prescriptions refilled at any pharmacy in their system. Many pharmacies even contact patients when their prescriptions need to be refilled. If customers request it, pharmacists will refill the prescription and have it waiting when the customer arrives.

Home delivery is another way pharmacies can enhance possession convenience. Pharmacies usually cannot afford the expense of free delivery, except for very important customers, but for a reasonable fee customers can receive items within a day or so through U.S. Mail or private package delivery companies.

It is not always possible for pharmacies to keep every product that patients may want. With so many expensive prescription products on the market, it can be prohibitively expensive to stock them all in sufficient quantities. The high carrying cost of prescription drug inventory forces most pharmacies to maintain tight inventories.

One solution is to dispense partial prescriptions and have the customer pick up the remainder at a future date. It is important that systems be in place to do this without breaking the law. Some pharmacies have been accused of purposely dispensing partially filled prescriptions, submitting the cost of the full prescription to third-party insurance companies, and pocketing the money when patients do not return to get the remaining portion of the prescription filled.[14]

Another solution is to maintain virtual inventories of a broad selection of products available for online purchase. Customers can order from a list of the business's products on the Web. Once a customer places an order, the marketer acts as a middleman and directs the manufacturer or other supplier to send the product directly to the buyer. Payment from the customer goes to the marketer, who then pays the supplier. Thus, there is no need to store products or manage physical inventory. In theory, the marketer can maintain an unlimited selection of products in virtual inventory. Amazon.com is a merchandiser well known for its use of virtual inventories.

To ensure that drug coverage plans do not impede possession convenience with cumbersome formulary policies, pharmacies need to work closely with pharmacy benefit managers. When a plan denies reimbursement for a prescription drug or some other problem occurs, it is important that a process be available for quick resolution. If the problem is not solved quickly, the patient is likely to be angry—and to blame the pharmacist.

Some pharmacies address possession convenience by limiting their services to specific target markets, such as people with certain diseases. Specialization permits pharmacists to offer a more comprehensive selection of products and services to a select group of patients. CVS has apothecary-style CVS ProCare pharmacies located across the United States.[15] These pharmacies provide specialized services for patients with complex or expensive drug regimens, particularly patients who are being treated for HIV/AIDS or with transplantation drugs or injectable biotechnology products. Many other retail chains have similar specialty pharmacies.

Transaction Convenience

Transaction convenience refers to the speed and ease with which a customer can complete a transaction. Customers who have completed their shopping and are ready to pay are often frustrated by long lines at the cash register. Transaction convenience can be increased in the following ways:

- Using self-service kiosks like those used by self-serve gas stations or automated teller machines.
- Enabling customers to run their purchases over a scanner and pay for them with a credit card, rather than wait for a clerk.
- Cross-training employees for different positions so they can fill in wherever needed.
- Permitting employees to make simple managerial decisions. Shifting decision-making authority to lower-level employees—for example, allowing a cashier to make simple decisions so that customers do not have to wait for managerial approval.
- Using robotics and automated dispensing devices to speed up the dispensing process.
- Improving daily workflow. Well-designed work areas can reduce wasted effort.

Conducting a Convenience Audit

Pharmacy employees and managers need to understand consumer perceptions of the convenience of their business. They need to see the pharmacy as consumers see it. Each pharmacist should be able to answer the following questions about the business:[13]

- How easy is it to enter the parking lot by foot and by car?
- How long does it take to get from the parking lot to the door?
- How long does it take to get from the door to the pharmacy department?
- What obstacles do customers face between the parking lot and the pharmacy department?
- How long is the wait at the pharmacy at different times of the day?
- How many times does the telephone ring before an employee answers it?
- How difficult is it to reach the pharmacist by telephone?
- How long does it take before the automated telephone answering system connects to a human being?
- How often does the pharmacy run out of stock?
- How often do customers ask for items the pharmacy does not stock?
- How many different ways can a patient reach a pharmacist?

In attempting to answer these questions, it is important for pharmacists to act as if they have never been in the pharmacy. For example, trying to maneuver through the store by using only the signage can help identify signs that are unclear and confusing.

RELATIONSHIP MARKETING

Relationship marketing is a strategic orientation or philosophy of business that focuses on keeping and improving business with current customers, rather than on acquiring new customers. This strategy assumes that customers prefer to maintain an ongoing relationship with one organization rather than switch among providers in search of greater value.

Businesses that practice relationship marketing usually find that it is much cheaper to keep current customers than to attract new customers, because current customers do not require promotional discounts or advertising directed toward attracting new customers. The concept of relationship marketing is compatible with pharmaceutical care, because pharmaceutical care is based on the development of a pharmacist–patient relationship.

Relationship marketers segment their market according to which customers are likely to become long-term customers. They do not try to attract customers who switch from business to business.

Relationship marketers further segment their customers according to profitability. Banks often practice relationship marketing by claiming it is unprofitable to keep customer accounts that maintain low dollar balances. Therefore, banks assess additional charges on all low-balance accounts, even accounts that have been maintained for years. Customers either pay the bank charges (and become more profitable) or leave (and the bank loses an unprofitable customer).

Benefits for the Patient

Since long-term relationships are less expensive for a business, savings can be passed on to customers in extra services or reduced prices. Money a pharmacy does not spend on advertising and promotion can go toward updating patient medication profiles or remodeling stores for patient counseling. Other benefits of maintaining relationships include the following:

- Searching for a good, reliable service provider is difficult and stressful. When a business meets the customer's needs, the customer is less likely to leave that business, because of the hassle of finding a replacement.

- Patients know what to expect. People like to know that when they visit a pharmacy, it will take a predictable number of minutes to have their prescriptions filled, that certain products will be available, and that parking will not be a problem.
- The pharmacist is able to meet the special needs of the patient. Many patients want their pharmacist to know them as a person—to know, for example, that they do not have children at home and do not like child-proof prescription containers. They like their pharmacist to remember what was discussed about their diabetes at the previous visit. They also like to know that the pharmacist knows them well enough to call them by name.

Benefits for the Business

Businesses can benefit from relationship marketing in the following ways:[16]

- As customers become satisfied with a company, they tend to spend more money each year with that company.
- Attracting new customers incurs advertising and other promotional costs, operating costs of setting up new accounts, and time costs of getting to know the customer. Sometimes these costs exceed the profits generated by a short-term customer. Studies have demonstrated that increasing customer retention by 5% can increase company profits by 35% to 95%.
- Loyal customers are likely to provide positive recommendations to friends and family. They are not likely to complain to others about occasional bad service. Word-of-mouth recommendations are much more effective in influencing purchasing behavior than any paid advertising.
- An indirect benefit of loyal customers is employee retention. It is easier for a firm to retain employees when the firm has a stable base of satisfied customers. Employees like to serve satisfied customers they know, rather than faceless, demanding customers. In turn, employees who are satisfied in their jobs provide higher quality services and have less turnover. This leads to greater profits for the firm.

The $100,000 Customer

Losing a customer can be very expensive to a company. A customer can easily spend $200 a month in the prescription department of a pharmacy. That works out to $2,400 of business per year. That customer may take maintenance medications and continue spending that much (or more) indefinitely. In 10 years, the customer will spend $24,000 in the prescription department and may spend an equal amount on front-end merchandise ($48,000). A happy customer will probably tell others, resulting in at least one more lifetime customer ($96,000). Therefore, losing a single customer can cause the company to lose $100,000 or more.

INNOVATION STRATEGIES

An innovation is any change in the marketing mix that customers perceive as new. It can be a change in products, services, or processes. Customer adoption of innovations depends on a complex mix of factors, including the relative advantage provided over competing products, the ease with which an innovation can be incorporated into the customer's life, and the perceived risk of adopting it.[17]

Innovations can be used to[18]

- Find new customers for the product (e.g., expand pharmacy services to customers with pets).
- Find new uses for a product (e.g., use Super Glue to close wounds).
- Increase usage of existing products (e.g., offer a customer loyalty card).
- Expand a product line (e.g., offer disease management in addition to basic dispensing services).
- Expand distribution intensity (e.g., increase the number of pharmacies in an area).
- Expand distribution over a wider geographic area (e.g., expand into new geographic markets).
- Penetrate the market position of competitors (e.g., develop a service that will draw away a competitor's target customers).

Innovation in Pharmacy

In pharmacy practice, the typical innovation is an incremental change, such as a new computer program, reorganization of the pharmacy layout, a coupon promotion plan, or a change in the work process. Many such changes are not really innovations, but imitations of other pharmacy businesses. Pharmacies can appear very similar in their marketing strategies. Most pharmacies have similar merchandise, services, layout, and overall atmosphere. The typical pharmacy strategy consists of some variation of low pricing and one-stop shopping convenience.

Lack of innovation in marketing strategies is common in many industries. Kim and Mauborgne[17] state that this is because competitors "share a conventional wisdom about who their customers are and what they value, and about the scope of products and services their industry should be offering." When a majority of businesses within an industry share the same conventional wisdom, they end up competing in essentially the same way.

A casual review of pharmacy trade magazines shows that most pharmacies follow a similar set of strategies: convenience, low price, emphasis on the pharmacist, merchandise variety, and niche marketing. As a result, they may have trouble differentiating themselves from their competitors.

Innovative marketing strategies can be risky. They require that companies change and establish new ways of doing business. This can be difficult to do, especially when the old way is still profitable. In addition, many new products and services fail on the market. For example, superstores selling durable medical products and adaptive equipment for home use have been slow to catch on.[19]

Identifying Innovations

With an open mind and good imagination, pharmacists can identify new market opportunities.[17]

Differentiate Yourself from Direct Competitors

Innovative pharmacists continually look for ways to differentiate themselves from competitors who offer similar products and services (*intratype competitors*, described in Chapter 2). Rather than mimicking innovations by their direct competitors, these pharmacists seek new ideas by identifying unmet needs.

Consider a pharmacy's direct competitors for filling patients' prescriptions. Patients can take their prescription to an independent, chain, grocery, or mass-merchandiser pharmacy. Or they can receive the medication from the physician's office, go to a drive-through pharmacy, fill the prescription through a mail order or Internet pharmacy, have the prescription transmitted to a pharmacy electronically or by telephone, or decide not to fill the prescription. All of these choices focus on the product—on getting the drug to the patient as quickly and cheaply as possible.

Rather than focus on direct competition for getting the drug to the patient, a pharmacy seeking to differentiate itself might choose to focus on the health care experience. Instead of aiming to get patients in and out as quickly as possible, the pharmacy could concentrate on being a desirable destination where people could explore health-related products and services. A pharmacy in Boulder, Colorado, has done this.[20] Pharmaca Integrative Pharmacy integrates natural remedies, herbal supplements, and alternative therapies with modern medical practices and prescription drug therapies. Shoppers are treated to light jazz or classical background music, scents from aromatherapy candles, and subdued lighting from strategically placed track lights. Contrast that with the typical community pharmacy that uses bright fluorescent lighting, Muzak, and a traditional merchandise mix.

Identify Indirect Competitors

Pharmacists looking for innovations can also get ideas from *inter-type competitors*, who compete indirectly by providing distinctly different products that meet similar customer needs and wants (see Chapter 2). Consumers choose products and services that they think will solve their problems. They are less interested in what is provided than in how well it meets their needs.

Consumers may consider products and services from many different industries to meet their needs. A person who is interested in an evening of entertainment might choose from the film, television, theater, restaurant, or sporting industries. Similarly, a person who catches a cold might choose chicken soup (food industry), cold medicine (pharmaceutical industry), echinacea (herbal industry), or a visit to a physician (medical services industry).

If pharmacists want to identify new solutions to patient problems, they must understand how consumers make these choices. Table 9-1 shows the steps involved in choices for treating a cold. Each choice results in different actions and outcomes. When patients go to a physician for a cold, they must make an appointment, go to the office, wait for the physician to become available, get a prescription or other treatment recommendation, go to a pharmacy, wait while the prescription is filled, and finally go home to take the medication. After going through this process, the patient may receive some symptomatic relief, but the cold will not resolve faster than with any of the other options.

Many people are too busy to visit a physician for a cold, so they choose self-treatment that may be as efficacious as a physician visit, without the time and expense. They might choose nonprescription medications, herbal products, or food.

Self-treatment carries its own risks. The patient may be suffering from a more serious condition that needs medical treatment. What might appear to be a cold could actually be pneumonia or some other serious infection. Self-treatment also carries the risk of adverse effects and interactions with prescribed drugs.

TABLE 9-1   Consumer Choices for Treating a Cold

Option	Steps	Outcome
Go to a physician	1. Make an appointment and go to the office. 2. Get a prescription. 3. Have the prescription filled at a pharmacy.	Significant time and effort spent. The condition resolves itself in approximately the same time as it would with other options. Some symptomatic relief possible. The patient is assured that the cold is not something else.
Choose a cold medicine	1. Go to a pharmacy or other store that stocks nonprescription medications. 2. Decide among various nonprescription choices.	Some time and effort required to go to the store. If the customer is unfamiliar with the choices, he or she must seek assistance from store personnel. The customer may be concerned about adverse effects or drug interactions. Some symptomatic relief possible.
Choose an herbal product	1. Go to a pharmacy or other store that stocks herbal medicines. 2. Decide among various herbal choices.	Some time and effort required to go to the store. If the customer is unfamiliar with the choices, he or she must seek assistance from store personnel. The customer may inappropriately feel safe from adverse effects and drug interactions.
Treat with food	1. Go to the kitchen cupboard. 2. Open a can of chicken soup.	Minimal time, effort, and money spent. May be reminded about how colds were treated during childhood and feel some comfort.

The patient's options have different costs and benefits. Pharmacists are in an excellent position to help the patient with the selection process. In fact, many already do. One study indicated that pharmacists make 6,108 recommendations for nonprescription drugs to patients each year.[21] However, pharmacists can do much more.[22] They can encourage patients to discuss their options. Patient–pharmacist communication can be enhanced if the pharmacist is readily available and on the lookout for consumers who are in need.

Communication can also be enhanced through good shelf displays. During cold season, the pharmacist can display a brochure or sign that delineates the most common options for treating a cold and the consequences associated with each option. The display could grab customer attention with pictures of a physician, a nonprescription medication, an herbal product, and a can of chicken soup above discussions of each option. Good displays can educate consumers about treatment alternatives and direct them to the pharmacist if necessary.

Provide Simpler Alternatives

Every day, health care consumers in the United States hear about complex and costly innovations for treating serious illnesses—advances that overshoot the needs of the vast majority of patients. Most patients' illnesses are uncomplicated and can be easily managed through basic diagnoses and treatments. Yet the dominant players in health care—educators, physician specialists, pharmaceutical companies, and hospitals—devote far less effort to finding simple, convenient, affordable means of meeting the needs of most patients than to developing highly sophisticated new treatments and technologies.

The overemphasis on high-tech, high-cost cures provides opportunity for disruptive innovations—the use of simpler solutions that meet most people's needs.[23] Examples include the substitution of nurse practitioners for general practice and specialty physicians, of patient self-care for physician-directed care, and of vaccinations at pharmacies instead of physicians' offices. Disruptive innovations compete by filling the gap left by businesses that focus on serving the profitable high-end market. They take advantage of opportunities to fill consumers' needs in less expensive ways.

Figure 9-6 illustrates disruptive innovations in patient care. The hierarchy of health care services increases in complexity from self-care providers (pharmacists, herbalists) to physician specialists (allergists, dermatologists). As specialists focus on treating the sickest patients, less highly trained providers can take on new roles. Family practitioners may perform diagnostic and treatment tasks formerly restricted to the domain of specialists. In turn, nurse practitioners and physician assistants manage conditions formerly managed by family practitioners. Drugs that were originally available only by prescription can now be purchased over the counter, along with self-diagnostic devices for diabetes, cholesterol, blood pressure, and pregnancy. The move toward consumer-directed health care and improvements in technology will continue to drive this trend.

Pharmacists have been participants in disruptive innovation. By selling and teaching about the use of self-treatment and self-diagnostic products, they have met the needs of patients who might have visited physicians' offices. In addition, pharmacists have provided immunizations,

FIGURE 9-6 Disruptive innovations in health care. Rx-to-OTC = switch from prescription to nonprescription status for a drug.

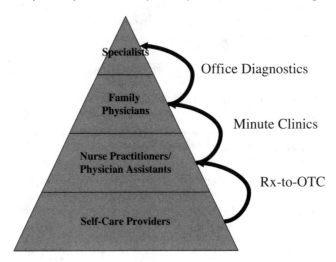

specialty medicine services, disease management, and a range of other services that were once the sole territory of physicians.

Pharmacists should realize, however, that disruptive innovations can compete with their practice. An example is dispensing machines in physicians' offices. Some patients may decide to sacrifice the value of pharmacist services for the convenience of one-stop treatment of their medical needs.

Consider Participants Other Than the End User

Ideas for innovations can come from thinking about participants other than the end user (i.e., the patient). Patients rarely make purchasing decisions about health care products and services without help from others (Table 9-2).

The patient may be the one who takes medication or receives treatment, but many times the decider is a physician, not the patient. The physician chooses a treatment for the patient, and the patient is expected to follow the physician's directions.

Third-party payers, such as insurance companies, employers, and the government, also influence treatment choice. Third-party payers may exert influence through co-payment policies, prior-authorization programs, and formularies. Other times, they act as deciders by refusing to pay for specific treatments.

TABLE 9-2 Participants in the Health Care Purchase Process

Decision-Making Role	Examples
End user	Patients
Decider	Physicians, patient, family members, payers, pharmacists, nurses, managed care plans, government (laws, rules), pharmacy benefit managers, employers and others who pay for health insurance
Influencer	Physicians, patient, family members, payers, pharmacists, nurses, pharmaceutical industry, managed care plans, wholesalers, government (laws, rules), pharmacy benefit managers, employers and others who pay for health insurance

Additional parties who may influence health care decision-making include nurses, pharmacists, employers, family members, and friends. Depending on the situation, they can take on a variety of roles in the purchase process. Pharmacists who understand the roles played by each party can identify new market opportunities.

The pharmaceutical industry has been very successful over the years in targeting different participants in the drug-use process. Companies no longer market prescription drugs solely to physician prescribers. They now promote pharmaceuticals to the public, advocacy groups, politicians, health care payers, and anyone else with a role in the process of purchasing drugs.

Pharmacists too have learned to target other participants in the drug-use process. In the past, they marketed their services almost exclusively to patients, because most patients paid for their medications out of pocket. The spread of prescription drug insurance and the resulting influence of managed care have forced pharmacists to cater to the desires of employer groups, pharmacy benefit managers, managed care companies, and physician groups. In some cases, the consequences have been negative: reduced dispensing fees. In other cases, positive outcomes have occurred: contracts with managed care providers to provide disease management services, and collaborative practice agreements with physicians to help them manage patient health conditions and control drug costs.

Each party involved in health care decisions has a different definition of value. Finding ways to serve these different customers can offer opportunities for pharmacists.

Add Value to the Drug-Use Process

Complementary or value-added products or services facilitate the appropriate use of medications. Dispensing services are a complement to physician prescribing, because they reduce the delivery of inaccurate and dangerous prescription drugs. Pharmaceutical care services complement basic dispensing, because they reduce drug-related problems.

Pharmacists can identify new opportunities to provide complementary services by first defining the total solution that customers seek when choosing a product or service. Although health is an important outcome of a pharmacy visit, it is not the only one. Many older, retired patients see a visit to the pharmacy as a social outing—an opportunity to get out of the house and chat about everyday matters. Some pharmacies encourage the use of the store as a social center by offering café sections or waiting areas where customers can catch up on local news and conversation.

Pharmacists can find new complementary service opportunities by considering what happens before, during, and after a visit to the pharmacy or other health care provider. It may be helpful to review Chapter 6, on the process of consumer decision-making. Opportunities that add value to the prescription drug process can be identified by mapping out all of the steps involved from the time of problem recognition to the time the medical condition is resolved. Consider the following questions:

- When and how do consumers realize they need physician services?
- When and how do consumers realize they need pharmacy services?
- Whom do they consult about their medical conditions?
- What media do they use for health information?
- When, where, and how do consumers decide to seek pharmacy services?
- What issues are important in selecting pharmacy services?
- What problems do consumers have in finding, purchasing, and paying for pharmacy services?
- What problems do consumers have once they have purchased pharmacy products or services?

Answering these questions can offer ideas for easing barriers in patients' drug-use process. Pharmacies can enhance problem recognition by creating displays that stimulate patients' curiosity about health topics. Pharmacists can do the same by engaging customers in conversations about health needs and interests. Pharmacies can have a section for health care books. Comfortable seating and even a coffee or snack bar can be provided to make the pharmacy an inviting, pleasant place to go. Pharmacists can improve postpurchase evaluation by inviting patients to discuss problems they have after leaving the pharmacy.

Add Emotional Appeal

Pharmacists usually promote the functional appeal of pharmacy goods and services—practical issues such as price, location, and quality—over their emotional appeal. On the assumption that people are thoughtful and rational in their actions, pharmacists highlight cognitive arguments about the utility and value of pharmacy products. But pharmacists may be missing an opportunity.

Other industries recognize the value of emotional appeals to consumers. Cosmetic companies successfully evoke a wide range of emotional images of their products, even though most cosmetics are made up of the same basic ingredients. It is often said that the cosmetics industry sells beauty and hope. If appeals were rational, much of the magic of cosmetics would be lost.

A company's emphasis on functional or emotional appeal sets customers' expectations of the business. Most pharmacies have trained their customers to expect speed, price, and location in the purchase of pharmaceuticals. Pharmacies could challenge the status quo by adding more emotion to the pharmacy shopping experience.

A great deal can be learned from the coffee industry. It has done a wonderful job of taking a functional product and injecting emotion into the consumption process. Functionally, coffee can be promoted on the basis of how hot it is, its freshness, and its cost. But Starbucks and other companies have made coffee drinking into a special event. Who ever would have thought that people would wait in line for the privilege of paying $5 for a steaming solution of coffee beans? Starbucks has changed the coffee shop from a place to buy a cup of coffee to a "caffeine-induced oasis."[17]

Some pharmacies tap into emotion. Those with soda fountains appeal to childhood memories. Other pharmacies emphasize the emotional bonds that exist between pharmacists, patients, and communities. Many small pharmacies appeal to emotions through the unique mix of merchandise they carry. Traditional merchandising rules might not recommend stocking craft supplies, gift items, and even deli supplies in pharmacies. However, sometimes a nontraditional mix of merchandise can help small pharmacies compete against large chains. Rather than being just a place to make purchases, they offer a unique shopping experience.

ETHICAL MARKETING STRATEGIES

Marketing practices that are seen as ethical can improve the image of a firm, enhance consumer trust, increase satisfaction, and make customers more likely to do business with the firm.[24] Marketers can use the following questions to assess the ethics of their strategies.

1. Would I be embarrassed to describe my actions to friends, family members, or professional colleagues?
2. How would I feel if a marketer acted in a similar manner toward me?
3. How would an objective jury of my peers judge my actions?
4. Does the strategy benefit my customers less than, as much as, or more than it benefits me?
5. Is the strategy consistent with our firm's mission and ethics code?
6. Am I taking advantage of a population that is vulnerable because of age, education, income, language, or some other factor?
7. Do consumers have sufficient knowledge to make a good decision?
8. Are consumers free to choose another provider if I do not serve them well?

SUMMARY

Pharmacists have traditionally relied on a limited number of strategies for marketing their services. This chapter presents several new strategies to consider.

References

1. Johannes L. Feisty mom-and-pops aim at drugstore chains. *Wall Street Journal.* March 20, 2000:A1.
2. Porter ME. *Competitive Advantage: Creating and Sustaining Superior Performance.* New York: Free Press; 1985.
3. Kubas L. Ten practical ideas for competing with Wal-Mart. *Can Bus Curr Aff.* 1996;4(6):13.
4. Posey LM. Competing with Sam's Club. *Consult Pharm.* 1992;7:497.
5. Medicine Shoppe has the Rx for success. *Chain Store Exec Shopping Center Age.* 1991;67(4):23–5.
6. www.medicineshoppe.com. Accessed October 27, 2006.
7. Buzzell RD. Competitive behavior and product life cycles. In: Wright JS, Goldstucker JL, eds. *New Ideas for Successful Marketing.* Chicago: American Marketing Association; 1966:46–68.
8. Cox WE. Product life cycles as marketing models. *J Bus.* 1967;40:375–84.
9. Jernigan JM, Smith MC, Banahan BF, et al. Descriptive analysis of the 15-year product life cycles of a sample of pharmaceutical products. *J Pharm Mark Manage.* 1991;6:3–36.
10. Wright RW. How Zantac became the best-selling drug in history. *J Health Care Mark.* Winter 1996:25–8.
11. Kotler P. *Marketing Management: Analysis, Planning, and Control.* 4th ed. Englewood Cliffs, NJ: Prentice Hall; 1980.
12. Wiederholt JB. Development of an instrument to measure evaluative criteria that patients use in selecting a pharmacy for obtaining prescription drugs. *J Pharm Mark Manage.* 1987;1:35–59.

13. Seiders K, Berry LL, Gresham LG. Attention, retailers! How convenient is your convenience strategy? *Sloan Manage Rev.* Spring 2000:79–89.
14. Ukens C. Fill 'er up. Drugstore chains pressing for partial-Rx fill standard. *Drug Top.* March 16, 1998;142:9.
15. ProCare helps build CVS brand. *Chain Drug Rev.* 2000;22(21):61.
16. Heskett JL, Sasser ED, Schlesinger LA. *The Service Profit Chain.* New York: The Free Press; 1997.
17. Kim WC, Mauborgne R. Creating new market space. *Harv Bus Rev.* 1999; 41(3):79–89.
18. Bradley F. *Marketing Management: Providing, Communicating and Delivering Value.* Upper Saddle River, NJ: Prentice Hall; 1995.
19. Ho R. Health care superstores go through some growing pains. *Wall Street Journal.* May 12, 1997.
20. Gentry CR. Health, harmony and higher sales. An ordinary drug store becomes an extraordinary health-and-wellness center. *Chain Store Age Exec Shopping Center Age.* 2001;77(4):41.
21. Cardinale V. Pharmacists as OTC counselors. *Drug Top.* 1994;138(13): S6–S9.
22. Morrow D. Improving consultations between health-care professionals and older clients: implications for pharmacists. *Int J Aging Hum Dev.* 1997; 44(1):47–74.
23. Christensen CM, Bohmer R, Kenagy J. Will disruptive innovations cure health care? *Harv Bus Rev.* 2000;78(5):102–12.
24. Ingram R, Skinner SJ, Taylor SA. Consumers' evaluation of unethical marketing behavior: the role of customer commitment. *J Bus Ethics.* 2005;62: 237–52.

Additional Readings

Doucette WR, Pithan ES, McDonough RP. Pharmacy service alliances: a tool to reduce uncertainty and create new revenue streams. *J Am Pharm Assoc.* 1999;39:697–702.

Holdford D. Disease management and the role of pharmacists. *Dis Manage Health Outcomes.* 1998;3(Jun):257–70.

McDonough RP, Doucette WR. Building working relationships with providers. *J Am Pharm Assoc.* 2003;43(5 Suppl 1):S44–S45.

Exercises and Questions

1. What problems might occur when pharmacists copy each other's marketing strategies?
2. What is an innovation? What are the benefits and costs of being highly innovative?
3. Porter suggests that there are three generic marketing strategies—cost leadership, differentiation, and focus. Which of these would be most appropriate for promoting your program or service?

4. Name one pharmacy service or merchandise item that you think is in each phase of the product life cycle: introduction, growth, maturity, and decline.
5. What is gained and lost when pharmacists adopt convenience strategies? Compare and contrast access, search, possession, and transaction convenience.

Activities

1. Go to an independent or chain pharmacy Web site. Write a short paragraph summarizing how the pharmacy positions itself in the market using various elements of the marketing mix (i.e., the four P's). What products and services make up its strategic portfolio? How would you describe its overall portfolio strategy?
2. Conduct a convenience audit of a pharmacy or other business that you frequent. Assess the access, search, possession, and transaction convenience of the business.

PART V

SEGMENTATION AND PROMOTION

CHAPTER **10**

MARKET SEGMENTATION

Objectives

After studying this chapter, the reader should be able to

❏ Define *market segmentation, targeting,* and *positioning.*
❏ Discuss the purpose of market segmentation.
❏ List characteristics of desirable market segments.
❏ List ways in which pharmacists can segment their markets, and give examples of each.
❏ Suggest several ways in which practicing pharmacists can conduct market research.
❏ Discuss the steps involved in segmenting markets.

A recent overview of the U.S. market for alternative therapies[1] discussed how segments of the market differed in their use of those therapies. Use differed by sex, geographic location, and personal circumstances. Women were more likely than men to use any alternative therapies, particularly aromatherapy, faith healing, and vitamins and herbal products. Geographically, people living in western states were most likely to use acupuncture or acupressure, go to chiropractors, and use massage therapy. Faith healing was most likely to be used in southern states, and aromatherapy in the Northeast. Residents of the Midwest were least likely to use any alternative therapies. Nationwide, people were more likely to use alternative therapies that were covered by health insurance or recommended by physicians. People were also more likely to use alternative therapies for conditions for which no clearly superior therapy was available.

Segmentation is a fundamental part of the marketing concept. Marketers realize that it is usually undesirable to try to serve all potential customers in a market, because each customer has different needs, wants, habits, and circumstances. The only way to satisfy everyone in a market would be to offer an infinite array of products and services at any time or place, free of charge!

Instead, marketers attempt to identify those individuals in the market who can be served most effectively and profitably. This process, called segmentation, is accomplished by categorizing individuals in the market according to shared characteristics, such as age, buying habits, or lifestyle. Those characteristics are used as a basis for developing a marketing mix that is targeted to groups' special needs, wants, and behaviors. This chapter explains why pharmacists need to segment their markets and discusses how they can do so.

Marketers use segmentation to identify similarities within groups of consumers and benefit from these similarities. Although every person in the world is different, it is still useful to group people according to consistent characteristics and make generalizations about these groups. Such generalizations can help marketers serve their customers better. Marketers who practice market segmentation are in a better position to

- *Identify opportunities in the market.* Opportunities exist when not all customer segments are served well. Segmentation helps identify poorly served, profitable segments of the population.
- *Tailor a unique marketing mix.* Segmentation permits the targeting of specific customer groups, to which a unique mix of price, product, promotion, and place can be offered.
- *Charge and receive higher prices.* A unique marketing mix can enhance customers' perceptions of value and allow higher prices to be charged.
- *Serve customers more efficiently.* Segmentation permits an organization to specialize. It can be more efficient to offer specialized services and products for only a few segments instead of maintaining the capacity to serve all customers.
- *Gain a competitive advantage.* Organizations that can identify market opportunities and offer a unique marketing mix can have an advantage over competitors.

In the past, segmentation was less important in the development of marketing strategy. In the mid-20th century, companies were able to meet consumer needs by using a mass marketing strategy—one that attempts to serve the entire market with the same marketing mix, offering every consumer the same price, location, promotion, and product mix. Because there was tremendous demand for products and services at that time, sellers who offered a uniform marketing mix to customers could succeed.

Today, mass marketing is no longer a useful strategy because there is too much competition for consumer demand. Pharmaceuticals now can be purchased at grocery stores, mass merchandisers, independents, chains, franchises, clinics, and physicians' offices. Drug products can be obtained through mail order, telephone, vending machines, drive-through pharmacies, and the Internet.

Marketers that use a mass marketing strategy to meet consumer needs now find it impossible to compete with marketers that practice segmentation. Competitors that use segmentation can lure away the most profitable segments of the mass market with unique promotional appeals, services, product features, and the like. Over time, the mass marketer is left with only the least profitable customers.

SEGMENTATION, TARGETING, AND POSITIONING

The terminology associated with market segmentation can be confusing. Segmentation is often referred to indirectly with terms such as target marketing, niche marketing, target groups, and demographics. When people use these terms, they are usually speaking of segmentation.

Market segmentation can be defined as dividing a market on the basis of differences and forming subgroups based on common characteristics. Individuals in markets can be segmented by sex, age, behavior, and other characteristics. Pharmacists may segment their patients by disease state; this is useful because knowing a person's disease state can help a pharmacist understand the amount and types of services that person might need.

Market segmentation goes hand in hand with *targeting* and *positioning*. Segmentation identifies variables that can be used to target desirable groups of individuals. A pharmacist who wants to serve the osteoporosis market can use sex and age as a basis of segmenting the market. Within the osteoporosis market, women over the age of 65 may be targeted, because they are at increased risk for fractures. On the basis of unique characteristics of this segment, a marketing mix can be chosen that clearly positions pharmacist-directed osteoporosis services in the minds of targeted customers. Pharmacists may attempt to position themselves in the minds of patients as "the drug expert" or "the most accessible health professional." Positioning is achieved through promotional communications, the merchandise and services offered, and other elements of the marketing mix.

IDENTIFYING DESIRABLE MARKET SEGMENTS

Segmentation is useful only if it provides some competitive advantage in serving customers. The challenge is to determine which customer segments are desirable. Desirable market segments need the following characteristics:

> *The value of segmentation lies in identifying segments that are more responsive to your targeted marketing mix than to those of your competitors.*

- *The segment must be identifiable.* It is easy to identify patients who fall into demographic categories defined by age, sex, and income. Other classifications may be difficult for most pharmacists to use. A segment labeled "hypochondriacs" would not be desirable if individuals in the segment were not easily distinguished from "non-hypochondriacs."
- *The segment must be accessible.* Pharmacists need to be able to reach each market segment with a customized marketing mix. Segments must be accessible both for the delivery of the product and for promotional communications. Using the hypochondriac example above, marketers would need to identify where individuals in the segment could be found, what media they are exposed to, and ways they could be easily reached and served.
- *The segment must be of sufficient size.* Customer segments must be large enough to be profitable to an organization. Since segments often require a customized marketing mix, the segment must have enough revenue-generating potential to cover the extra costs associated with customization. Thus, current and future revenue associated with each segment must be estimated.
- *The segment must be responsive to your targeted marketing mix.* The value of segmentation lies in identifying segments that are more responsive to your targeted marketing mix than to those of your competitors. If a targeted mix cannot satisfy the market segment better than the mix offered to the general market, then segmentation provides little advantage.

SELECTING SEGMENTATION VARIABLES

Segmentation variables are used as surrogates for behavior. Knowing a patient's age and disease state is useful in segmentation because these variables are associated with levels of prescription drug use. Segmentation variables should be chosen on the basis of their relationship to the behavior in which you are interested.

Selecting variables to use in segmenting markets can be relatively simple. Much of the information needed for segmentation already exists in customer databases or in a marketer's personal knowledge of customers. Segmentation becomes difficult only as more complex multivariate analyses of the market are conducted. Pharmacists can choose segmentation variables in several ways:

- *Through experience and intuition.* Pharmacists often rely on personal experience and judgment to identify and evaluate customer segments in a market. Most experienced pharmacists have a good idea of the needs, tendencies, and characteristics of their patients.
- *By adopting the ideas of others.* Professional pharmacy organizations (e.g., American Pharmacists Association, American Society of Health-System Pharmacists, National Association of Chain Drug Stores, and National Community Pharmacists Association) and publications such as *Drug Topics, Pharmacy Times,* and *U.S. Pharmacist* present interesting ideas about segmenting the market for pharmacy services and products. Pharmacists can often find ways to apply these ideas to their settings.
- *By analyzing customer data.* Pharmacists can analyze data collected from prescription records, customer databases, and consumer surveys, as well as data purchased from market research companies, to select segmentation variables. The key is to analyze the information in a way that provides unique insight into behaviors of individuals within specific market segments.

EMPIRICAL VERSUS HYPOTHESIS-DRIVEN APPROACHES

A segmentation approach can be empirical or hypothesis driven. In empirical segmentation, the marketer's choice of segmentation variables is based on professional experience or information collected from the literature. This approach resembles empirical treatment by physicians (i.e., making clinical decisions on the basis of professional knowledge). Pharmacists might use empirical segmentation to classify patients by disease state, frequency of drug use, and age—characteristics that have well-known associations with the need for pharmaceutical care.

In hypothesis-driven segmentation, the marketer tests hypotheses about the relationships between market segmentation variables (e.g., demographics, benefits sought) and outcomes (e.g., utilization, sales, adherence). The purpose is to gain insights about actual and potential customers that can be used to secure a competitive advantage.

Hypothesis-driven segmentation builds on information used in empirical segmentation, such as the opinions of managers and published information. However, it goes further by relying on market research techniques to identify patterns of consumer behavior. These techniques can include qualitative research (e.g., focus groups, personal interviews) as well as multivariate research methods (e.g., conjoint analysis, logistic regression, structural equation modeling). Pharmacists with good people skills and common sense may be able to conduct their own focus groups and personal interviews. For multivariate research, pharmacists usually contract with marketing research firms or universities. It is common for researchers at universities and contract research organizations to analyze demographic, drug-use, and insurance plan information to identify variables that help predict drug utilization patterns.

Both empirical and hypothesis-driven segmentation methods have advantages and disadvantages for marketers. Empirical segmentation relies on the marketer's experience and ability to understand which variables are useful. This experience is gained from reading business and professional publications and conducting business every day. It is only as expensive as the amount of time devoted to it and the cost of the subscriptions to publications. It is a time-tested method; business owners have relied on their intuition and knowledge to serve customers for thousands of years.

The problem with empirical segmentation is that life in today's world is so complex. Managers are bombarded daily with tremendous amounts of information about customer behavior and the actions of competitors. Even if they are able to keep up with all of the insights offered in business and professional publications, this may not provide an advantage, since competitors have access to the same information. Managers often find it useful to get help in identifying patterns of behavior that will offer a competitive advantage.

Hypothesis-driven segmentation uses methods from a variety of fields to gain greater understanding of consumer behavior and markets. Marketers borrow from psychology, sociology, anthropology, computer science, economics, communications, and other fields to propose and test hypotheses about markets. The methods can be as rigorous as anything found in medicine or the basic sciences.

In general, the more rigorous the methods used in hypothesis-driven segmentation are, the higher the cost. Thus, larger companies or professional associations are more likely to use this type of research. Nevertheless, smaller firms can conduct simple hypothesis-driven research on current and potential customers. An independent pharmacist could use patient profiles to identify utilization data associated with patients' requests for help with their medications. The pharmacist might hypothesize that greater numbers of medications, changes in therapy, specific disease states, and specific age groups are associated with requests for help. The pharmacist could then test whether these variables can consistently predict requests for help. If so, specific patients who might need greater pharmacist assistance could be targeted.

MARKETING STRATEGIES ASSOCIATED WITH SEGMENTATION

Segmentation is used to implement either differentiation or focus marketing strategies (described in Chapter 9). A company that uses a differentiation strategy selects two or more segments for targeting. Companies that use this approach attempt to select a portfolio of products and services to meet the needs of multiple customer groups. A pharmacy may choose to target seniors, customers motivated by convenience, and diabetes patients. To meet the needs of all of the segments, a broad promotional mix is required.

Focus strategies target market niches. A niche is a small, narrowly defined market. Marketers that use niche strategies select a single, profitable segment that offers the best opportunity for success. Ideally, marketers should choose niches that are (1) large enough to be profitable, (2) underserved or ignored by competitors, and (3) able to be exploited by the unique skills and capabilities of the marketers.

Figure 10-1 shows how the osteoarthritis market might be segmented by using differentiation, niche, and microniche strategies. Osteoarthritis patients could be grouped into those with mild, moderate, and severe osteoarthritis and according to method of payment: Medicaid, private insurance, and self-pay. A differentiation strategy might target the self-pay and Medicaid markets, with elements in the marketing mix specific to patients in each segment. Although the pharmacist will continue to serve the untargeted private insurance segment, no special effort will be made to meet the needs of this segment.

Alternatively, a more focused, niche strategy might aim to serve only self-pay patients. A microniche strategy might even limit efforts to the mild osteoarthritis, self-pay market.

A common assumption is that a business's largest segment should be targeted, but this strategy is not always the most appropriate. The largest patient segment for many pharmacies is made up of patients who want fast and cheap drugs with minimal services. The competition for this segment is often fierce, and its contribution to profits can be slim, especially if third-party insurance reimbursements are low. Pharmacists may find

FIGURE 10-1   Segmenting the osteoarthritis market using differentiation, niche, and microniche strategies.

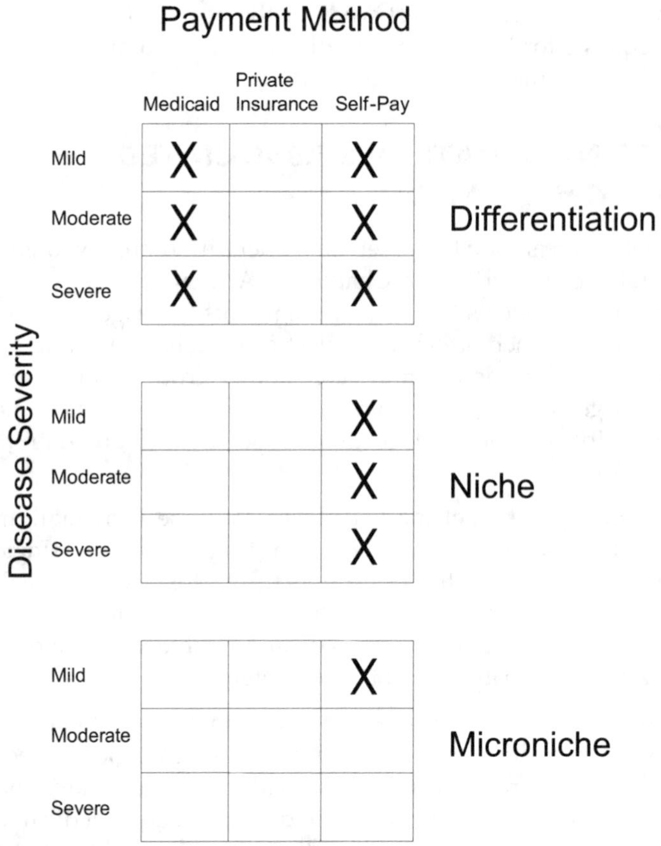

Payment Method

	Medicaid	Private Insurance	Self-Pay	
Mild	X		X	
Moderate	X		X	Differentiation
Severe	X		X	

	Medicaid	Private Insurance	Self-Pay	
Mild			X	
Moderate			X	Niche
Severe			X	

	Medicaid	Private Insurance	Self-Pay	
Mild			X	
Moderate				Microniche
Severe				

Disease Severity

it more profitable and satisfying to target smaller, more lucrative segments such as pediatric patients with chronic diseases or women at risk for osteoporosis.

DEMOGRAPHIC SEGMENTATION

The most common ways of segmenting markets are demographic, geographic, psychographic, behavioral–utilization, and benefits segmentation (Table 10-1). Markets are most easily segmented according to demographic and geographic categories. Demographic variables such as age, sex, income, and ethnicity can be used to subdivide the market. Demographic data about consumer markets are widely available from numerous public and private sources (Table 10-2), many of which can be accessed on the Internet.

TABLE 10-1 Common Ways of Segmenting Markets

Basis of Segmentation	Segmentation Categories	Examples
Demographic	Age, sex, family size, income, occupation, education, family life cycle, religious affiliation, nationality	Family life cycle: newlywed, married with young children, married with older children, empty nesters
Geographic	Country, region, metropolitan statistical area, city, county, state, neighborhood, rural	Region: Northeast, Midwest, Northwest, Southwest, Southeast
Psychographic	Personality, lifestyle, values	Lifestyles: health hermits, recluses, ailing outgoers, health indulgers
Behavioral	Actual behavior: frequency of use, situations, user status, loyalty, adoption of innovations Potential behavior: readiness to buy or act Mixed behavior: variables at risk for drug-related problems	Willingness to adopt innovations: innovators, early adopters, early majority, late majority, laggards
Benefits	Benefits sought are varied and almost endless	Quality buyers, service buyers, value buyers, economy buyers

TABLE 10-2 Sources of Demographic Data for Pharmacists

U.S. Bureau of Labor Statistics
U.S. Census Bureau
U.S. Department of Commerce
U.S. Internal Revenue Service
U.S. Social Security Administration
National Center for Health Statistics
Individual state and local government sources
Small Business Administration
Professional and trade associations and journals
American Demographics magazine
Prevention magazine
Local chambers of commerce
Local libraries

The federal government provides a wealth of health statistics and demographic data. Census data available on the Internet at www.census. gov contain demographic information including sex, age, race, Hispanic origin, household type, housing occupancy, homeowners, renters, school enrollment, educational attainment, marital status, disability status, labor force status, commuting, occupation, income and benefits, and poverty. Census data are often too general for individual businesses. More detailed demographic data can be purchased from private market research companies and local chambers of commerce.

Demographics constitute one of the most common bases of segmentation, because it is easy to classify people according to age, sex, and other demographic variables. Furthermore, consumer behavior is often linked to demographics. For instance, women use health care services and prescription drugs more frequently than men do.[2] Women also know more about health matters, are more likely to seek health information, and more frequently use preventive care and nonprescription medications.[3]

Demographics are useful in developing targeting strategies. Knowing the age and makeup of households (e.g., sex, marital status, number of children) can help pharmacists target key decision makers in the selection and administration of prescription drugs. Data on the average income in a neighborhood can indicate consumers' available resources. Information about the percentage of full-time workers in an area can give insight into the amount of time customers have available for shopping and health care.

The Senior Segment

Health care providers have given much attention to the market for older Americans. The senior market segment is one of the greatest users of prescription medications and other forms of health care. Seniors make up 13% of the population but consume more than 30% of all prescription drugs and 25% of nonprescription medications.[4] They are the fastest-growing age segment of the population and have the highest average discretionary income of any age group.[5] For these reasons, health care providers have found the senior market an attractive one to target.

However, several problems are associated with segmenting the senior market.[5] One problem is defining the age at which a person is considered a "senior." Marketing researchers have used ages ranging from 50 to 65 years to define the lower end of the senior market. Another problem is that there is not a single senior market segment; seniors make up multiple age segments. Seniors who fall within specific age ranges (e.g., 55 to 64, 65 to 74, 75 to 84, and 85 and over) are more likely to be similar than seniors of all ages. To further complicate matters, people of similar chronological ages may have different physical, psychological, and social ages. Many people do not look or act their age. Seniors with debilitating diseases can appear to be much older than their chronological age, while healthy, active individuals can appear to be much younger. Some seniors may act young, while others may act older than their age.

Literature on the topic indicates that age should not be the sole variable for segmenting the senior market. Bone[5] identified five variables that have been recommended for segmenting the senior market:

- Discretionary income (the amount of money available for spending after paying for rent, utilities, and other fixed expenses),
- General level of health,
- General activity level,
- Amount of discretionary time not taken up with family, job, and social activities, and
- Degree of social interaction with others.

Cohort Segmentation

Another way of segmenting consumers by age is to divide them into cohorts. A cohort is a group of people of the same generation; the same historical events during formative periods of their lives have shaped their personalities and behaviors.[6] Members of each cohort share common core values and behaviors. People who lived through the Great Depression are likely to be thrifty. Those who came of age during the Vietnam War are likely to challenge authority. Depression Babies, the Silent Generation, the Swing Generation, the Greatest Generation, Baby Boomers, Generation Jones, Baby Busters, Echo Boomers, Generation X, Generation Y, and Millennials are names given to generational cohorts. Table 10-3[7-9] describes some cohorts with increasing needs for pharmacist services and pharmacy products.

GEOGRAPHIC SEGMENTATION

Geographic segmentation permits pharmacists to target patients on the basis of location. It can be used to locate lucrative market segments and target those segments with promotional communications. Geographic information is most useful when linked to other segmentation variables such as age, sex, and spending levels.

The U.S. Census Bureau and organizations such as local chambers of commerce provide demographic and other data that can be linked to geographic location. Pharmacists looking for a potential pharmacy location can go online and find data on consumers by location, income, age, and other demographic variables. Competitor locations can be plotted, along

TABLE 10-3 Comparison of Generational Cohorts

Variable	World War II Generation	Post-War Generation	Baby Boomers I and II
Year of birth	1922 through 1927	1928 through 1945	1946 through 1965
Description	As these people came of age, they were unified by the shared experience of a common enemy and a common goal. They became intensely romantic and developed a strong sense of self-denial that outlived the war.	These are the war babies who benefited from a long period of economic growth and relative social stability.	Born after World War II, they were pampered as children and developed a strong sense of entitlement. Disparaged as the "me generation," they feel that they should have it all.
Celebrity members	Paul Newman, Betty White, Maria Callas, Sammy Davis Jr., Bob Barker, Dick Van Dyke, Jimmy Carter, Charlton Heston	Robert Duvall, James Earl Jones, Elvis Presley, Jesse Jackson, Bob Dylan, Rush Limbaugh, Woody Allen	Bill and Hillary Clinton, George W. Bush, Rosie O'Donnell, Bill Gates, Madonna, Michael Jordan
Money motto	Save a lot, spend a little.	Save some, spend some.	Spend, borrow, spend.
Music	Swing	Frank Sinatra	Rock and roll
Marketing profile	They are frugal and want value. They have relatively positive attitudes.	Financially conservative, but willing to spend on themselves. They have a lot of money. They grew up respecting experts as role models. They want information from knowledgeable sources.	Many distrust authority. They want to hear from peers who use the products. Juggling careers, children, and elderly parents, they want products and services that save time and make life easier.

Sources: References 7–9.

with local traffic patterns. Market and economic analyses of the area can also be acquired. Much of this information is available free of charge or for a nominal fee.

Additional geographic data can be purchased from market research firms. Holubiak[10] used data from IMS America, a major provider of prescription drug data, to describe prescription drug use by geographic area. Prescribing data were linked to metropolitan statistical areas to identify variations in drug use. The research showed a sevenfold variation in per capita spending on cholesterol-reducing drugs among different parts of the United States. Prescribing patterns in geographic locations were found to be related to drug company sales efforts, provider-to-population ratios, and the relative number of physician specialists.

Another study used demographic data to determine the rural distribution of primary care physicians, pharmacists, and other health care providers.[11] This research was conducted to identify markets underserved by health care professionals. Computer-based linking of ZIP Codes and provider practice information identified opportunities for pharmacists in many rural areas to provide clinical services such as blood pressure and glucose monitoring and patient education.

PSYCHOGRAPHIC SEGMENTATION

For answering many marketing questions, demographic and geographic data have limited usefulness. These data cannot explain why consumers act the way they do. Age, race, and sex tell little about why a person might select one product over another or be more susceptible to certain promotional messages. To better understand these issues, marketers conduct psychographic research.

Psychographic segmentation is based on the premise that consumer behaviors are influenced by personality, lifestyle, and values. Psychological and sociological research methods, including surveys, focus groups, and personal interviews, are used to identify consumer values, beliefs, and attitudes. Psychographic segmentation is useful for shaping promotional strategies, for product development, and for communication decisions.[12] There are numerous ways to segment markets psychographically.

Personality Segments

Personality segments are based on behavioral traits or personality characteristics such as compulsive, controlling, conservative, socializer, extrovert, and need to achieve. Although heavily studied, personality has not been found to be a consistent predictor of consumer behavior.[13]

Lifestyle Segments

Lifestyle can overlap with personality characteristics but is more useful for segmentation.[14] Lifestyle relates to the activities, interests, and opinions of consumers. Lifestyle segmentation reflects a group's priorities and beliefs about various issues. People's actions (e.g., purchases) tend to be consistent with their interests and opinions.

Lifestyle segmentation has been used to classify senior populations. In 1993 Moschis[15] grouped the 53 million adults in the United States 55 years of age and over into four segments: health hermits (20 million), frail recluses (8 million), ailing outgoers (18 million), and health indulgers (7 million). It was found that these segments could be used to target senior preferences for products, payment methods, and responsiveness to promotional efforts. Shufeldt et al.[16] used lifestyle to identify differences in seniors' nonprescription purchasing behavior. They segmented seniors as follows: family oriented (25.6%), young and secure (19.4%), active retiree (18.1%), self-reliant (20%), and quiet introvert (18.9%). Using these segments, they were able to identify differences in the perceived importance of price, commercial influences, and personal influences on purchases of nonprescription medications.

Table 10-4[17] illustrates how lifestyle segments can be used in contacting and communicating with patient groups. Patients were divided into five segments—disciples, medical buffs, naturalists, immortals, and fatalists—on the basis of their approach to health care. Each segment's characteristics and barriers to treatment can be used to tailor marketing messages and communication methods.

Segmentation by Values

Values segmentation attempts to identify values upon which people base their lives and day-to-day actions. Values associated with consumer purchasing behavior include self-respect, security, excitement, sense of fun and enjoyment of life, having warm relationships, self-fulfillment, sense of belonging, sense of accomplishment, and being well respected.[18]

Knowing which values are important to customer segments can help marketers design and deliver their messages. A pharmacist who wants a patient to adhere to a medication regimen might communicate a different message for a segment that most values security than for a segment that values fun and enjoyment of life.

TABLE 10-4 Marketing Segments by Approach to Health Care

Segment	Characteristics	Barriers to Treatment	How to Reach	Message
Disciples	Obedient, trusting, and highly compliant with therapies	Sometimes forgetful	Pharmacists, advertising, popular press	Remind; reinforce benefits of treatment
Medical buffs	Engaged, adherent; trust physicians but feel in control of own health	Have strong brand ideas; first to switch brands	Internet, medical publications, brand-specific ads	Position treatment as patient–physician relationship; stress brand superiority
Naturalists	Shun pharmaceuticals in favor of holistic remedies	Distrust traditional treatments; anxious about side effects	Guerrilla marketing, condition-specific Web site, nonbranded ads, point-of-purchase displays	Position treatment as part of healthy lifestyle; emphasize the natural
Immortals	Devil-may-care types; disregard physician's recommendations	Ill-informed; often in denial	Family members, peers, telephone reminders	Deliver wake-up call; clarify necessity for treatment
Fatalists	Feel health is out of control; often noncompliant	Feel hopeless and helpless	Family members, peers, telephone reminders	"With help, you can overcome symptoms"

Source: Adapted with permission from reference 17.

Psychographic Research and Drug Use

Psychographic studies have segmented users of pharmaceuticals. In one study of users of cold remedies, four different market segments were identified:[19]

- *Realists* are not overly concerned with protection but are not fatalistic either. They view remedies positively and consider nonprescription therapies to be a convenient health care solution.
- *Authority seekers* are neither fatalists nor stoics about their health. They prefer some stamp of authority on remedies, from either a physician or a pharmacist.
- *Skeptics* have a low concern for health and are the least likely to use medications, including cold remedies.
- *Hypochondriacs* are very concerned with health matters and regard themselves as prone to being affected by all germs and diseases. These people tend to take medications at the onset of the first symptoms of a cold. They seek the expertise and authority of a health care provider for reassurance.

Piepho[20] used psychographic segmentation to identify consumers who might be less compliant with medications. Three groups were identified: dissatisfied, energetic, and sedentary. People in the dissatisfied segment were unhappy with several aspects of health care, including their physician, the drugs prescribed for them, and the cost of drugs. They were more skeptical of medical advice given and less likely to be compliant. In contrast, patients in the energetic segment were active, positive, and optimistic. They were more satisfied with most aspects of their health care and the most compliant of the three groups. People in the sedentary segment had good relationships with their physician and were highly satisfied with care but were less likely to be involved in their therapy. As a result, they were less compliant than energetics but more compliant than dissatisfieds. Strategies for improving compliance in each group were provided.

COMBINING PSYCHOGRAPHIC AND DEMOGRAPHIC VARIABLES

Some researchers combine demographic and psychographic variables to segment markets. Morris et al.[21] segmented users of the AARP (formerly American Association of Retired Persons) pharmacy service into four types of information seekers. "Ambivalent learners" perceived themselves as less than totally healthy and likely to seek out further information about their health and medicines. "Uncertain patients" perceived themselves to be less knowledgeable about their health conditions but in actuality were no less knowledgeable than others. They also believed that adherence to medication regimens would be difficult. "Risk avoiders" used medical information-seeking as a risk-control coping strategy. "Assertively self-reliants" did not feel much need for medical information.

BEHAVIORAL SEGMENTATION

Most individual pharmacists do not have the background in psychometrics, the research skills, or the funding to use psychographic segmentation. Pharmacists may find value in grouping patients into categories based on perceptions and lifestyles. However, a method that is more accessible and easier for the average pharmacist to apply is behavioral segmentation.

Behavioral segmentation uses information about consumer actions and choices to group customers. In a health care environment, it often deals with utilization of health care services and products. Behavioral segmentation criteria might include the type of health insurance or health plan choices available, the frequency of visits to health care providers, self-care habits, prescription drug use, nonprescription and herbal medication use, preventive care behaviors, and level of participation in pharmaceutical care activities. Many marketers believe segmentation based on actual behavior is particularly valuable because of the strong relationship to future behavior.[14]

One argument for using behavioral segmentation in health care is that a relatively small number of people use a disproportionate amount of health care services and products. This phenomenon is described by the *Pareto principle*, which states that approximately 80% of most problems can be attributed to roughly 20% of their potential causes. The Pareto principle would suggest that pharmacists should target the 20% of the market associated with drug misuse, health care spending, and other behaviors, because the potential positive impact will be disproportionately greater than the marketing effort. The following examples show the 80–20 rule at work in health care:[22]

- Ten diagnostic categories accounted for approximately 75% of all medical expenditures in 1987.
- For one large employer, 33% of asthma patients accounted for 73% of the costs of treating the disease. Thirty-seven percent of patients with chronic obstructive pulmonary disease accounted for 86% of the costs.
- Infants make up less than 6% of all children up to 18 years of age but account for 24% of the spending.
- Arthritis and back or spine problems account for 40% of all disabilities in the United States.

Three types of behavioral segmentation are of interest to pharmacist marketers. The first is associated with actual behavior related to the use of products and services. The second is associated with potential behavior related to the likelihood of use. The last, a mix of the first two, considers both actual and potential behavior.

Segmentation Based on Actual Behavior

Usage

Consumers are often segmented according to the frequency with which they use products and services. Studies by market research firms such as Mediamark classify usage of a variety of consumer products (e.g., cough and cold medicines) and services (e.g., physician visits) by light, medium, and heavy users. Some of the products and services studied by Mediamark are listed in Table 10-5.[23]

TABLE 10-5   Products and Services Market Researchers Have Classified by Usage

Asthma relief remedies (nonprescription)	Hemorrhoid remedies
Athlete's foot remedies	In-home pregnancy tests
Cold, sinus, allergy remedies	Incontinence products: used in past 6 months
Condoms: bought in past 6 months	Indigestion aids and upset stomach remedies
Contact lens cleaning/wetting solutions	Lactose-intolerance products
Cough drops (nonprescription)	Laxatives
Cough syrup (nonprescription)	Medicated throat remedies
Denture adhesives and fixatives	Nasal sprays
Denture cleaners	Pain-relieving rubs and liquids (nonprescription)
Diarrhea remedies	Premenstrual or period pain remedies
Dieting, diet pills (nonprescription)	Prescription drugs: used in past 12 months
Dieting, meal supplements	Sleeping tablets (nonprescription)
Dieting, methods	Smoking cessation products/services
Dieting, reasons	Stimulants (nonprescription)
Doctor visits	Sunburn remedies
Eye wash and drops	Suntan and sunscreen products
Eyeglasses, contact lenses, and sunglasses	Toothache, gum, and canker sore remedies
Eyewear, prescription: where purchased	Vitamin and mineral supplements
Groin irritation remedies	Wart and corn removers
Headache remedies and pain relievers	

Source: Reference 23.

Heavy users are often targeted by marketers, in the belief that persuading one heavy user to use a product or engage in a behavior is better than persuading three or four light users.[24] In pharmacy, disease management services are based on this belief. *Disease management* is a type of health care intervention directed toward populations of patients who have medical conditions that are especially expensive to the health care system. It is believed that attracting patients with diabetes or asthma to a pharmacy will generate greater sales and lead to a greater reduction in overall health care costs than will attracting several people with minor illnesses.[25,26] *Case management* is also based on usage. Case management attempts to help individual patients with severe health problems navigate efficiently through the health care system. It usually targets individuals who have multiple, chronic, costly conditions.

Heavy users may be a desirable target market, but there are times when targeting moderate or light users or nonusers is better. A large number of patients who are light users or nonusers of health care can indicate latent, unmet demand. Patients who rarely use pharmacist services may actually be those who most need them (e.g., patients who are noncompliant with medications). Their lack of usage may be due to unawareness of their personal pharmaceutical needs, unfamiliarity with the benefits of pharmacist services, or financial or physical barriers to receiving services.

Occasion

Patients can also be grouped according to the occasions or situations in which they make purchasing decisions. Gehrt and Pinto[27] found that consumer selection of pharmacists, physicians, and other health care providers depends on the individual consumer's situation. Consumers were asked to rate the appropriateness of health care choices (e.g., physician, emergency room, pharmacist) in (1) treating major and minor illnesses, (2) at home and on vacation, and (3) for the respondents themselves or for treating family members. The respondents indicated that for major illnesses at home, physicians and emergency rooms were the best alternatives. For major illnesses away from home on vacation, consumers preferred urgent care centers in addition to physicians and emergency rooms. For minor illnesses at home or on vacation, consumers considered the pharmacist, medicine cabinet, chiropractor, and "do nothing" alternatives to be equally appropriate. There was no difference in responses according to whether treatment was being considered for the respondents themselves or for family members.

User Status and Loyalty

Other behavioral segments address user status and consumer loyalty. User status refers to previous use. It might consider whether consumers are

FIGURE 10-2 Segmenting customers according to their tendency to adopt innovations.

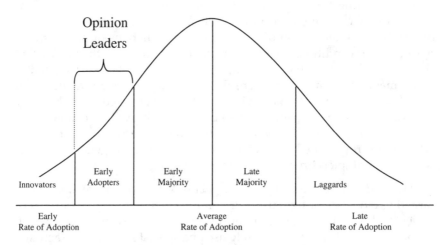

first-time users, former users, repeat users, or potential users. This classification is useful for pharmacists because knowing past use can be helpful in selecting marketing strategies designed to influence future use. Loyalty to a product or service is also a common way of segmenting customers. Marketers often treat customers who have been consistently loyal over time differently from those who have demonstrated partial or no loyalty.

Willingness to Adopt Innovations

Behavioral segmentation can also classify individuals according to their innovativeness and the speed at which they adopt innovations (Figure 10-2).[26,28]

Innovators are the first to adopt new ideas and products. They usually account for a small percentage of the population (approximately 2.5%). They are characterized as venturesome, eager to try new things, and willing to take risks. They have a broader viewpoint than the typical person, greater education, and the financial capability to absorb failures.

Early adopters are socially connected and influenced by innovators. They typically make up 13.5% of the population and are more likely to influence opinions than any other adopter category. They are sought out for advice, respected by others, and willing to share new ideas through word-of-mouth discussions.

Individuals in the *early majority* are influenced by early adopters, but they are careful, deliberate, and willing to take more time in making decisions. They make up approximately 34% of the population. Although not typically opinion leaders, they are usually well integrated socially.

Late majority individuals make up 34% of the population and are considered cautious and skeptical with regard to innovations. They tend to wait to adopt innovations until social and economic pressures force them to do so.

Laggards make up the last 16% of the population. They are traditional in outlook and look to the past in their decision-making. They are often socially isolated and resist innovations.

This behavioral segmentation scheme shows that adoption of innovations starts with a few individuals. Those innovators share their experiences with others until, over time, the innovation is spread widely throughout the population.

Marketers like to identify early adopters within a market. Early adopters are known as *opinion leaders* or *thought leaders* because they are socially connected and likely to influence the diffusion of innovations within a market. Because of their social connections, they are more influential than innovators. Drug companies commonly identify physician thought leaders and work to persuade them to try newly marketed drugs on their patients. The hope is that these thought leaders will adopt the drugs and encourage other physicians to try them.

Segmentation Based on Potential Behavior

A common method of segmentation by potential behavior is to group individuals according to their readiness to buy or act in some desirable manner. Marketers have divided buyer readiness into the following stages: unaware, aware, interest, evaluation, trial, usage, and repeat usage.[29] Knowing the stage of readiness a consumer is in can help improve the effectiveness of marketing interventions. Someone who is unaware or uninterested will likely require a different marketing mix than those in other readiness stages.

Pharmacists often segment patient populations according to readiness to act. One of the most common smoking cessation strategies is based on patients' readiness to change smoking behavior. The five stages of the transtheoretical model of change (described in Chapter 6) are used: precontemplation, contemplation, preparation, action, and maintenance. Individuals in the precontemplation and contemplation stages require different appeals and strategies than people in the later stages of readiness to act.

Segmentation Based on a Mix of Actual and Potential Behavior

In some cases, a combination of actual and potential behaviors is used to segment consumers. Koecheler et al.[30] developed a set of indicators to identify ambulatory pharmacy patients at increased risk for drug-related problems. The following indicators of actual and potential behavior were used to segment their patient population:

1. Patients taking 5 or more medications in their current drug regimen.
2. Patients taking 12 or more medication doses per day.
3. Patients whose medication regimen has changed four or more times in the past 12 months.
4. Patients who have more than three concurrent disease states.
5. Patients who have a history of noncompliance.
6. Patients who are taking drugs that require therapeutic drug monitoring.

Patients with these characteristics were more likely to have drug-related problems. Segmenting patients in this way can help target those patients who might benefit most from pharmacist intervention.

BENEFITS SEGMENTATION

Benefits segmentation groups customers according to the specific benefits they seek. It is especially useful for marketers because behavior is closely linked to the benefits sought.[14] Some consumers choose their pharmacy on the basis of convenience, because they want to simplify the search or minimize travel time. Others choose pharmacies because of the relationship with their pharmacist or the service received.

Segmenting customers according to benefits is consistent with the total product concept (described in Chapter 2), in which customers purchase the core benefits provided by products, not the tangible product. People purchase products and services to meet many different needs and wants—psychological, social, spiritual, and physiological. The marketer can identify and use benefit segments to better serve customers.

On the basis of benefit seeking, pharmacists might group their customers as follows:[29]

■ Quality buyers, who seek the best products and services without regard to cost.
■ Service buyers, who look for personal and caring services.

- Value buyers, who hunt for the best value for the money and expect service to match the price.
- Economy buyers, who favor the cheapest alternative.

Consumers of preventive health services have been segmented according to benefit seeking.[31] In-depth interviews of consumers found the following six benefit segments:

- *Hypochondriac.* People in this segment need and actively seek reassurance that they are healthy. They tend to overuse health services because they believe that doing so will improve their health. They are good customers for vitamins, self-diagnostic kits, and preventive therapies; by using these products, they think they are doing the right thing to maintain health.
- *Health seeker.* Health seekers strive for a long, healthy life and use preventive care as a means to that end. They actively participate in health behaviors such as exercise, healthy eating, and avoidance of smoking, illicit drugs, and alcohol. They actively seek information about healthy practices and preventive services such as health screenings and vaccinations. They also respond to the marketing of health foods.
- *Band-Aider.* Band-Aiders like to brag about how healthy they are. They take great pride in how little they have needed to use health care services. Preventive health care is undesirable to them because it directly contrasts with their self-image of robust health. Band-Aiders seek care only when they are very ill or injured.
- *Do not bug me.* People in this segment use negative health behavior such as overeating, smoking, and drug and alcohol use to cope with the daily stresses of life. They avoid preventive health care, although they may be the segment most likely to benefit from it.
- *Follower.* Followers seek the guidance of others for preventive practices. They might seek advice from friends, family members, or health care professionals. They tend to do what others recommend but can be skeptical that preventive health care will bring about the promised improvements in health. They are more likely to put off health care until they get sick. They are unlikely to use vitamins and preventive remedies or to attend health screenings unless it is recommended by others.
- *Self-sufficient.* These independent, self-reliant individuals tend to be skeptical of traditional health care and prefer to treat themselves with home remedies and nonprescription medications. Their skepticism often comes from previous negative experiences with health care.

SEGMENTATION FOR THE PRACTICING PHARMACIST

It is important for pharmacists to remember that the goal of segmentation is to help identify and predict consumer tendencies to act in specific ways. This information can then be used to influence consumer behavior in some manner. The value of segmentation variables is their ability to act as surrogates for behavior. The information has little value to a marketer if it cannot be put to use to predict and influence behavior.

> *The goal of segmentation is to help identify and predict consumer tendencies to act in specific ways. This information can then be used to influence consumer behavior.*

Researching the Market

In order to segment a market, pharmacists need to conduct research into their patients' needs and wants. There are several marketing research methods that any pharmacist can use, many of them at little or no cost.

Talk with patients. One-to-one conversations provide insight into customer needs. Good pharmacists talk with patients about their lives and problems to help identify better ways to serve them.

Invite a group of patients to chat about pharmacy services. This can be done in a formal focus group or less formally with a group of people sitting around a table. In focus groups, people are encouraged to share information they might not share in one-to-one conversations. Pharmacists can pay marketing research companies to conduct focus groups, or they can conduct them on their own. Before doing so, pharmacists might want to read up on focus group techniques to learn how to enhance the effectiveness of information collected.[32]

Conduct surveys. Surveys are useful for gathering information and statistics about a large group of customers. One problem with surveys is getting people to respond to them. The key to increasing the response rate is to make it easy to respond. Surveys should be as short as possible, easy to read, and accessible. Many businesses place customer surveys on 5 by 10 inch cards and locate them near the point of service. Pharmacists interested in conducting surveys can find numerous publications discussing how to do so.

Read the pharmacy and health care literature. There are many articles describing important trends, new developments in the profession, and ideas for segmenting patient populations.

Use the Internet. Internet search engines such as Google and Netscape permit pharmacists to search the world for information without leaving their chairs.

Mine patient data files. Pharmacists can analyze patient purchasing and usage patterns through scanner data or patient medication profiles. The data can be used to identify behavioral patterns that might be of use in marketing.

Observe how customers shop. Answer the following questions: What do they do while waiting for services? What do they purchase? How do they purchase? How much time do they take? On what components of the package or promotional material do they focus?

Test-market ideas. Before offering a service on a full time basis, hold a one-day event to test whether customers like the service and what they like or dislike about it. Consider expanding it to one day each week or full-time at one store in a chain.

Using Segmentation in Practice

Individual pharmacists can use segmentation to target specific customer groups for their services. Here are the steps:

1. Identify key market segments within your practice. Start with easy- to-define segments such as customers with different disease states, large numbers of prescriptions, or specific needs. As experience is gained, new segments may be identified.
2. Learn as much as you can about the segments in which you are interested. Try to identify how information in the published literature relates to your patients.
3. Describe a typical person in a market segment. Try to characterize how this person typifies the segment and what makes him or her different from those in other segments. This description is important in developing targeting strategies.
4. Determine the desirability of each segment. This can be done by calculating the average lifetime value of customers in the segment, the number of customers in the segment, or some other measure.
5. Select those segments on which you wish to focus and create a written plan for each segment. Describe what specific actions will be taken to meet the needs of customers in each segment.
6. Establish a budget for each segment. The budget should include allocations of both money and time. Explicit understanding of the costs involved will help improve the chances of success.

7. Develop measures for the success of targeting efforts (e.g., sales volume, number of repeat visits).
8. Choose a future date when you will reassess your marketing efforts.

SUMMARY

It is important to choose segmentation variables carefully. Select only one or two segmentation criteria to begin with; more than a few can be hard to keep track of. Make certain that the segments are based on clear marketing objectives and a solid knowledge of your customer base.

References

1. Fetto J. Quackery no more. *Am Demogr.* January 2001:10.
2. LaFleur EK, Taylor SE. Women's health centers and specialized services: segmentation strategies can be effective in targeting some female health care consumers. *J Health Care Mark.* 1996;16(3):16–24.
3. Aging boomers, new medicines draw men into health spotlight. *Drug Store News.* 2000;20(11):CP24.
4. Roller K. Pharmacists face challenge of surging elderly population. *Drug Store News.* September 21, 1998:CP1.
5. Bone PF. Identifying mature segments. *J Serv Mark.* Winter 1991;5:47–60.
6. Smith JW, Clurman A. *Rocking the Ages.* New York: Harper Business; 1997.
7. Gen,er,a,tion. *Richmond Times Dispatch.* April 2, 2001:B1.
8. Rice F. Making generational marketing come of age. *Fortune.* June 26, 1995; 131:110–3.
9. Meredith G, Schewe C. The power of cohorts. *Am Demogr.* December 1994; 16:22–31.
10. Holubiak M. Local area market dynamics. *J Manag Care Pharm.* 1988;4: 115–20.
11. Knapp KK, Paavola FG, Maine LL, et al. Availability of primary care providers and pharmacists in the United States. *J Am Pharm Assoc.* 1999;39: 127–35.
12. Morgan C, Levy D. To their health. *Brandweek.* 1998;35(3):30–3.
13. Bradley F. *Marketing Management: Providing, Communicating and Delivering Value.* Upper Saddle River, NJ: Prentice Hall; 1995.
14. Nylen D. Segmentation of markets. In: *Marketing Decision-Making Handbook.* Englewood Cliffs, NJ: Prentice Hall;1990:G-121–G-127.
15. Moschis GP. Gerontographics. *J Consum Mark.* 1993;10(3):43–53.
16. Shufeldt L, Oates B, Vaught B. Is lifestyle an important factor in the purchase of OTC drugs by the elderly? *J Consum Mark.* 1998;15:111–24.
17. Lam MD. Psychographic demonstration. *Pharm Exec.* 2004;24(1):78–83.
18. Kahle LR, Beatty SE, Homer P. Alternative measurement approaches to consumer values: the list of values (LOV) and values and lifestyles (VAL). *J Consum Res.* 1986;13(3):405–9.

19. Ziff R. Psychographics for market segmentation. *J Advert Res.* 1971;11(2): 3–9.

20. Piepho RW. Prescription for Compliance: Results of a Psychographic Study of and a Review of Recent Methodologies. Bridgewater, NJ: Hoechst Marion Roussel; 1997.

21. Morris LA, Tabak ER, Olins NJ. A segmentation analysis of prescription drug information-seeking motives among the elderly. *J Public Policy Mark.* 1992;11:115–25.

22. Herzlinger R. *Market Driven Health Care.* Reading, Mass: Perseus Books; 1997.

23. Mediamark Research Inc. Product summary reports. Available at: www. mediamark.com. Accessed October 25, 2006.

24. Wansink B, Park SB. Methods and measures that profile heavy users. *J Advert Res.* 2000;40(4):61–72.

25. Holdford DA, Kennedy DT, Bernadella P, et al. Implementing disease management in community pharmacy practice. *Clin Ther.* 1998,20(2):1–12.

26. Holdford D. Disease management and the role of pharmacists. *Dis Manage Health Outcomes.* June 1998;3:257–70.

27. Gehrt KC, Pinto RB. Assessing the viability of situationally driven segmentation opportunities in the health care market. *Hosp Health Serv Admin.* 1993;38:243–65.

28. Nylen D. New product adoption. In: *Marketing Decision-Making Handbook.* Englewood Cliffs, NJ: Prentice Hall; 1990:G-69–G-73.

29. Kotler P. *Marketing Management: Analysis, Planning, and Control.* Englewood Cliffs, NJ: Prentice Hall; 1980.

30. Koecheler JA, Abramowitz PW, Swim SE, et al. Indicators for the selection of ambulatory patients who warrant pharmacist monitoring. *Am J Hosp Pharm.* 1989,46:729–32.

31. John J, Miaulis G. A model for understanding benefit segmentation in preventative health care. *Health Care Manage Rev.* 1992;17(2):21–2.

32. Hassell K, Hibbert D. The use of focus groups in pharmacy research: processes and practicalities. *J Soc Admin Sci.* 1996;13:169–77.

Exercises and Questions

1. What is the purpose of segmenting pharmacy markets? Compare and contrast segmentation, targeting, and positioning.
2. List the characteristics of a desirable market segment.
3. Comment on why pharmacists may not want to target the largest segment in markets.
4. What demographic variables in Table 10-1 are most associated with prescription drug use in general? Oral antibiotics? Birth control products?
5. What problems are associated with targeting the senior market? What other variables within the senior market are useful in segmentation? How might these variables affect drug consumption and use?

6. How might an understanding of psychographics help pharmacists design promotional messages to different patient market segments?
7. What is the Pareto principle? How does it relate to behavioral segmentation?
8. Should pharmacists target light or heavy users of prescription medicines? Why?
9. Should pharmacists segment patients for pharmaceutical care according to disease state or general health care needs (i.e., case management)?

Activities

1. Go to www.sric-bi.com and take the VALS survey. What personality segment do you fall into according to the survey? How does your segment differ from classmates?
2. Divide potential customers for your product or service into different demographic, geographic, behavioral, and benefits segments. On the basis of characteristics of desirable market segments (page 212), select the segments that you wish to target, and justify your choice.
3. Visit the Web sites of professional associations and publications and identify at least one resource that discusses a potential segmentation variable.

11

MARKETING COMMUNICATION

Objectives

After studying this chapter, the reader should be able to

❑ Discuss the purpose of promoting pharmacy products and pharmacist services.

❑ Explain barriers to effective marketing communication, using the communication model.

❑ Describe the information processing model.

❑ Use the information processing model to discuss the relative effectiveness of various communication media.

❑ List the six forms of promotion used to communicate marketing messages.

❑ Explain the advantages and disadvantages of each of these forms of promotion.

❑ Offer basic recommendations for promoting services.

❑ Describe the steps used in developing a promotional plan.

If you're trying to persuade people to do something, or buy something, it seems to me you should use their language, the language in which they think.

David Ogilvy,
founder of the advertising network Ogilvy & Mather[1]

Communication is an essential component of the marketing mix. Marketers must communicate with consumers to inform them about their products, persuade them to use the products, and remind them to continue doing so. Without marketing communication, even a highly desirable,

well-priced, and convenient product can fail.
Marketing success requires communication
about the product's existence, features, price,
location, and benefits.

Promotion is communicating a message to prompt some immediate or future action by the consumer.

For effective communication, a marketer
must establish a clear image of the product in
the eyes of the customer. This involves asking,
"What value am I providing to my custom-
ers?" To answer this question, the marketer needs to have a clear definition of the product being promoted.

The marketer also needs an explicit understanding of the target market. Effective communication begins with a fundamental understanding
of the receiver. This includes insight into which customer segments would
benefit most from the product offered. Those segments can then be targeted for communications tailored to their interests and capabilities.

Not too long ago, pharmacists and other professionals debated
whether the use of advertising and other promotional methods was
unprofessional. Some pharmacists still say that promotional communications cheapen the profession. But this debate is no longer relevant, because
the market has made the decision. Promotional communications by professionals, including physicians, lawyers, dentists, and pharmacists, are
now widely accepted. The issue of whether to promote has been replaced
by how to promote.

The main messages promoted by pharmacies and pharmacy organizations are the value of pharmacy services and the image of pharmacists as
caregivers.[2] Television advertising and other media are used to highlight
the value of the patient–pharmacist relationship. This differentiates pharmacists by promoting their professionalism and the assistance they offer
to users of pharmaceuticals.

This chapter discusses the psychology of promotion and strategies
used to communicate with consumers. It describes how to design and
deliver effective marketing messages.

PROMOTION

Promotion is any type of communication designed to inform, educate,
or persuade customers about products.[3] At its most basic, promotion is
communicating a message to prompt some immediate or future action by
the consumer (Figure 11-1). Marketing communication can inform ("Prescription refills now on the Internet!" "Immunizations will be offered
from 10 am to 12 noon on Saturday"), persuade ("Our prices can't be beat!"

FIGURE 11-1 Elements of promotional communication.

Promotion   Consumer   Action

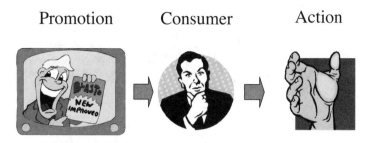

"Our employees care about you"), or remind ("Don't forget! We're still America's most trusted"). The goal of an individual message depends on the marketing situation.

Everything pharmacists do sends a message to the public. The image of the profession is shaped by our words and actions. Whether that image is what we want depends on how we define and transmit our message.

There is plenty of room for improvement in the way pharmacists promote their image. Critics have argued that pharmacists have done a mediocre job of defining their image in the customer's mind.[4–6] We may be among the most trusted professions, but the public has only a vague idea of what pharmacists actually do.

The current image of pharmacists is of our own making. Pharmacists often let others (e.g., the media) define our image rather than taking an active role in its management. Instead of educating patients about pharmacists' professional responsibilities, we let patients draw their own conclusions about what goes on behind the counter. The profession's negligence in promotion has left too many people today with an outdated image of pharmacists as pill pushers.

THE COMMUNICATION MODEL

To understand marketing communication, it is important to understand how consumers process the massive amount of information to which they are exposed. This includes how messages are sent, received, processed, and stored in memory. Familiarity with some simple models can help pharmacists maximize the effectiveness of their messages.

Whether the message is to inform, educate, or persuade, all communications follow a common model (Figure 11-2). A sender (the marketer) has a message for a receiver (the consumer). The sender of the message must encode the message in words or images. The message (e.g., "Buy our product") may be in pictures, written words, spoken words, sounds,

FIGURE II-2   The communication model.

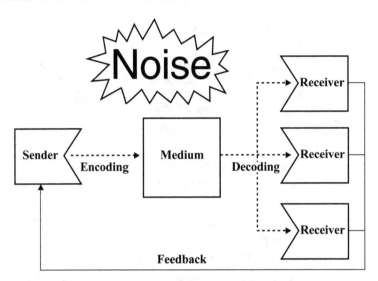

or symbols. The encoded message must be transmitted through some medium, such as television, radio, magazines, billboards, the Internet, or conversation. That message, under the right conditions, is then received and decoded (i.e., interpreted) by the receiver. Decoding of the message is influenced by factors such as the consumer's attention, attitudes, knowledge, and biases. In some cases the message received will prompt the receiver to act (e.g., buy the product). In many other cases the message is not acted on immediately and is either stored in memory for access at a later date or forgotten. All messages are transmitted in an environment full of the noise from thousands of other messages.

Many things can go wrong in the path represented by the communication model. The message may be poorly conceptualized, vague, or confusing. The desired receiver may miss the message, hear or see it incorrectly, interpret it wrong, or remember it inaccurately. With mass media (e.g., television or radio) communications, the problems are multiplied. A single message is sent to thousands or millions of receivers whose levels of sophistication, accessibility, and motivation are different, resulting in numerous interpretations of the same message. The message "Eat healthy food" can be perceived differently by people of diverse backgrounds and circumstances.

Marketing communication is complicated by the fact that we live in an age of "sound-bite decision-making."[7] People spend less time processing messages than they did in the past. The ever-increasing amount of information to which people are exposed has forced them to deal with information superficially. Multitasking is common; people simultaneously watch TV, talk on the phone, surf the Web, and juggle other activities. Consumers are likely to skim promotional messages, gather bits and pieces of data, and incorporate the data into some understanding that may be broad but not deep. To successfully compete for the consumer's attention, marketing messages about products and services must be available, clear, consistent, and coherent.

This is why marketers often use segmentation to develop unique promotional plans for different target populations. The goal is to find a promotional message and medium appropriate for each target market. Each market segment should receive a message geared to its level of interest, knowledge, and attention.

THE INFORMATION PROCESSING MODEL

Promotional communications face stiff competition for consumers' attention. The average person is exposed to 1,600 commercial messages each day.[8] Eighty of these are consciously noticed, and only 12 provoke some form of reaction. The difficulty in getting consumers' attention causes some marketers to do whatever it takes to be noticed, including placing their messages on almost anything (e.g., urinals, people's bodies, food products), anywhere (e.g., in movies and television shows, schools and public buildings).

Even when consumers do notice a promotional message, it may not be perceived in the way the marketer intended. In many cases, consumers distort the message so that they hear what they want to hear. In other cases, consumers lack the time, knowledge, or ability to interpret the message correctly.

Pharmacists who wish to enhance the effectiveness of their promotional communications need to understand how consumers process information—how they receive it, interpret it, and store it in personal memory. The information processing model in Figure 11-3 is useful in understanding consumer decision-making and designing communication plans. Between the sender and the receiver's response are five steps:

1. *Exposure.* The first step in marketing communication is to expose the receiver to the message. This requires selecting a medium that will get the message to the target receiver.
2. *Attention.* Next, the message must capture the attention of the receiver. The medium should be able to provide the message in a way that appeals to the interest of the receiver and can compete with the thousands of other messages people are exposed to daily.

FIGURE 11-3 The information processing model.

```
┌─────────────────────────────────────┐
│          Message Sent               │
│   through a Promotional Medium      │
└─────────────────────────────────────┘
                  │
┌─────────────────────────────────────┐
│       Exposure to the Message       │
└─────────────────────────────────────┘
                  │
┌─────────────────────────────────────┐
│       Attention to the Message      │
└─────────────────────────────────────┘
                  │
┌─────────────────────────────────────┐
│    Comprehension of the Message     │
└─────────────────────────────────────┘
                  │
┌─────────────────────────────────────┐
│     Acceptance of the Message       │
└─────────────────────────────────────┘
                  │
┌─────────────────────────────────────┐
│  Retention of the Message in Memory │
└─────────────────────────────────────┘
                  │
┌─────────────────────────────────────┐
│ Action Taken in Response to the Message │
└─────────────────────────────────────┘
```

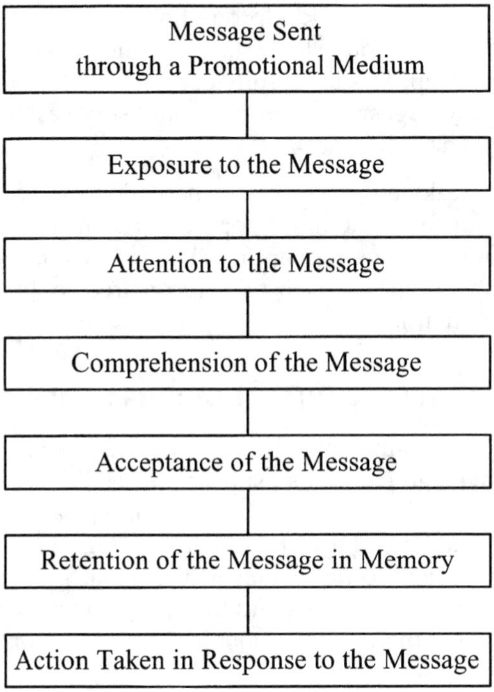

3. *Comprehension.* Attention then needs to lead to comprehension of the intended message. There are many ways to misunderstand a message. Comprehension depends, in part, on the receiver's motivation, knowledge, and biases. It is best for the message to be simple, vivid, and clear.
4. *Acceptance.* Messages that are clearly communicated and comprehended are not necessarily accepted. Many smokers clearly understand antismoking messages but do not accept them.
5. *Retention.* Even messages that are accepted are often forgotten. Messages need to be memorable. Humor or imagery can be used to establish the message in the receiver's mind. Repetition can also reinforce the image in memory.

In the information processing model, messages must progress through several stages before they can reach a consumer's memory. Only messages that are committed to memory can be acted upon. To be effective, the message must reach the consumer, grab his or her attention, be understood, be accepted, and be remembered. Failure at any stage of the model means ultimate failure of the communication.

> *To be effective, the message must reach the consumer, grab his or her attention, be understood, be accepted, and be remembered.*

Pharmacists can use this information processing model to evaluate the effectiveness of different messages in influencing the actions of customer groups. For example, the effectiveness of the following communication methods for influencing physician prescribing practices could be evaluated:

- Educational brochures directed to "Occupant,"
- Personalized letters to individual physicians to accompany printed educational materials,
- Patient-specific lists of prescribed medications,
- Continuing-education (CE) programs during lunch at a physician's office, and
- Face-to-face conversations with clinical pharmacists or other physicians.

Each of these communication forms has advantages and disadvantages. Educational brochures and personalized letters are inexpensive to produce and mail but are largely ineffective in influencing physician behavior.[9,10] The effectiveness of printed materials is low because physicians often do not read them. Materials may be screened by a secretary or thrown out unopened by the physician. Even when they are read, printed materials may be only superficially scanned for relevant information. Thus, printed messages frequently fail in the exposure or attention step of the information processing model. Personalizing the message with the physician's name or specific patient prescribing information may increase attention somewhat, but comprehension, acceptance, and retention of printed information usually are still low, so the message has relatively little impact on prescribing behavior.[9,10]

Oral communication of messages through CE programs might be expected to achieve greater levels of attention and comprehension than print media. CE programs tend to attract people who are interested in the subject matter and more receptive to the messages being communicated. However, interaction between the speaker and the audience often is low, and drifting audience attention may diminish the acceptance and retention of the message. The effectiveness of CE programs in influencing physician prescribing is small at best.[9]

The most effective form of communication for influencing physician prescribing is face-to-face conversation. This is commonly referred to as *academic detailing* or *counterdetailing*.[9,10] The term academic detailing originated with prescribing interventions at teaching institutions. The term counterdetailing is used because these interventions were initially designed to counteract information provided to physicians by pharmaceutical sales personnel (called detailers). Face-to-face communication, unlike print material, cannot easily be ignored. Comprehension and acceptance are enhanced because the message can be tailored to the interests and understanding of the physician. Retention of the message is reinforced because the presentation is more interactive.

Electronic systems offer further opportunity to influence prescribing. They enable pharmacists and others to communicate with physicians at the point of prescribing. Physicians can be informed, persuaded, and reminded through targeted messages, personalized educational interventions, updates, and electronic consultations. Relevant information can be provided when it is needed, in a way that is hard to ignore. Communications can be individualized to be more engaging and acceptable to physicians and thus more likely to be understood and acted upon.

PROMOTIONAL METHODS

In communicating their messages to targeted audiences, marketers use various methods of promotion that can be divided into two categories: *marketer controlled* and *marketer influenced* (Figure 11-4). In marketer-controlled methods, the message, medium, and delivery are directly managed through monetary payment. Advertising, personal selling, direct marketing, and sales promotions are marketer controlled; compensation is paid to the person or entity that delivers the message (e.g., the salesperson or advertising firm). In contrast, promotional methods that are marketer influenced do not involve quid pro quo compensation from the marketer to the entity delivering the message. Instead, marketers indirectly influence the messages through what are called *third-party techniques*. The strategies employed here separate the message from the self-interested messenger (i.e., the marketer);[11] they include public relations and word-of-mouth ("buzz") communications.

Marketer-Controlled Methods

Advertising, personal selling, direct marketing, and sales promotions differ in how they communicate marketing messages. Differences include the number of people likely to be exposed to the message (this is termed *reach*), cost per person reached, and level of impact on consumer behavior.

FIGURE 11-4 Forms of marketing promotion.

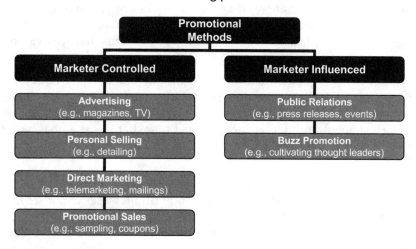

The advantages and disadvantages of each method are described in the following sections.

Advertising

Advertising is any paid, nonpersonal presentation promoting ideas, goods, or services.[3] It includes print messages (e.g., in newspapers, magazines, newsletters, outdoor ads, and Yellow Pages), broadcast messages (e.g., television, radio, podcasting), and Internet advertising (e.g., Web site banners).

Advertising in large newspapers or on radio or television is likely to be out of the financial reach of small pharmacy operations. However, small businesses can take advantage of a variety of low-priced, local advertising media, such as telephone Yellow Pages advertisements, business directory listings, fliers posted on bulletin boards in community buildings and businesses, advertisements in programs of community and high school theater groups, and penny-saver newspaper advertisements.

In addition to being less expensive, advertisements in local media may be perceived as more personal than those in major media such as television and magazines. Another advantage is that consumers tend to search local media for solutions to their problems. They are more likely to look at bulletin boards or in the Yellow Pages to find local businesses to serve their needs.

Some marketers argue that different strategies should be used for promoting merchandise than for promoting services, since product-oriented advertising sells things and service-oriented advertising sells performance.[12] It is relatively simple to advertise things, because tangible products can be easily represented in pictures or verbal descriptions. Advertising performance is more difficult. For instance, how does one characterize pharmaceutical care in an image or words that are clear and easy to understand?

Television news broadcasts often attempt to illustrate pharmaceutical services by linking pharmacists to something tangible. Many news stories about pharmacy show pharmacists counting tablets on a tray. The tablets are a convenient prop for letting viewers know that this is a pharmacist. Without seeing the tablets, viewers might not recognize the person as a pharmacist.

The unique characteristics of services, such as intangibility and inconsistency, make it difficult to convey meaningful messages about services in advertising. It is much easier to give consumers a vivid image of a product than of a service experience. Table 11-1 suggests strategies for advertising services.[13–15]

One strategy is to make services more tangible in ads. This might be achieved through images of physical facilities or use of concrete symbols or language. Seeing the counseling or drive-through area of a pharmacy gives consumers context for thinking about the service experience. Such images attempt to relate an abstract concept (i.e., a service) to a tangible one (i.e., an object).[13] Tangible objects associated with pharmacy services include computers, telephones, prescription bottles, and company logos.[15] Even a picture of a smiling pharmacist can be used. The mortar and pestle, a symbol of pharmacy's past, is still seen.

Another strategy is to make the relationship between the consumer and the provider explicit in the advertisement. Many pharmacy ads show a patient and a pharmacist consulting about medication. This gives consumers a clearer image of the service. Other ads show consumers speaking on the telephone (presumably to the pharmacy) or contacting pharmacies by Internet.

Documentation can be used in advertisements to underscore the quality and value of services. Using documented measures of quality helps differentiate one service provider from the next. Advertisements can highlight customer satisfaction scores or special awards for exemplary services. The Verified Internet Pharmacy Practice Site seal is awarded by the National Association of Boards of Pharmacy to Internet pharmacy sites that meet certain requirements. Consumers can use this symbol to identify quality Internet pharmacies.

Another way of emphasizing the quality and value of services in ads is to simulate word-of-mouth recommendations by showing people discussing

TABLE 11-1 Strategies for Advertising Pharmacist Services

Problem	Strategies
Services are intangible. Accordingly, services are more difficult to grasp conceptually.	Make pharmaceutical services more tangible in the advertisement. Incorporate physical elements of the service into the ad. Show a picture of the counseling area or the drive-through pharmacy. Associate the service with a concrete symbol.
Services are inseparable from their production and consumption. Services usually require the presence and participation of the customer.	Demonstrate the patient's participation. Show the pharmacist and patient together in the advertisement. Show the patient accessing pharmacist services by telephone or Internet.
Services are heterogeneous; no two service experiences are alike. Excellent service one day may be replaced by a horrible experience the next day.	Use documentation of the consistent high quality of pharmacist services. Include results of satisfaction surveys or Gallup polls in the ad. Display achievements such as certification as a diabetes educator or as a Verified Internet Pharmacy Practice Site. Simulate word-of-mouth recommendations with a testimonial from a customer about excellent service.
The service experience is difficult for consumers to visualize.	Show the service experience as a series of events. Illustrate superior pharmacy service in a television advertisement (e.g., when a pharmacist prevented a serious drug reaction). Include text that shows the simple steps involved in completing a telephone refill.

Source: References 13–15.

the services. This can be accomplished by having customers, real or simulated, talk about previous service experiences. Sometimes celebrity spokespersons are used. It is important that the celebrity in advertisements be seen as credible, likable, and representative of the image promoted by the marketer. Former Olympic gymnast Mary Lou Retton was used by Revco (now part of the CVS pharmacy chain) in its advertisements. She was probably chosen because she was likable and energetic and seemed trustworthy.

Finally, the steps involved in the service experience itself can be illustrated in advertising text or images. A visit to a pharmacy might be illustrated with a series of images showing a pharmacist receiving a prescription, checking the patient profile, calling the physician to verify information, and then giving the patient the medication, along with counseling.

Personal Selling

Personal selling is any oral presentation to customers as individuals or groups.[3] As a promotional method, it differs from advertising because it permits two-way communication. It is also the one promotional method engaged in by every pharmacist. Personal selling activities in pharmacy include patient counseling, telephoning physicians to get them to change a patient's therapy, giving hospital in-service presentations for nurses, participating in hospital grand rounds, having brown bag meetings, and academic detailing.

Pharmacists may not like having their patient and professional interactions characterized as personal selling—as sales promotion instead of health promotion. This concern relates to the word "selling." A better word might be "consultation." Consultation is consistent with the concept of modern personal selling, which emphasizes long-term relationships that serve the customer and discourages short-sighted tactics to promote quick sales.[16] Good personal selling helps customers use the product effectively, efficiently, and in a way that maximizes benefits over time—goals consistent with pharmaceutical care.

A five-step process for personal selling has been described by McDonough and Doucette.[17] Their model consists of an interactive exchange between the pharmacist and patient in which the information communicated becomes increasingly specific. The goal of the process is to identify how patients' needs can be satisfied.

- *Preliminary stage: Gather patient information.* In an exploratory session, the salesperson and customer introduce themselves to each other and decide whether there is sufficient interest and need to continue with the sales process.
- *Step 1: Assess information.* The salesperson moves beyond the general information exchange in the preliminary stage to more specific inquiries that can clarify the patient's needs and concerns. Using active listening techniques and open-ended questions, the pharmacist attempts to involve the patient in the search for a solution to his or her health care need.
- *Step 2: Ask probing questions.* The pharmacist asks more focused questions about specific patient needs. Patients are asked for precise information about the situation (e.g., What medications are you taking?

What health conditions do you have?), problems (e.g., Have you experienced any side effects? Are you able to control your blood pressure?), and implications (e.g., Are you able to be productive at work? Do you understand what will happen if you can't control your blood pressure?). Given this information, the pharmacist has patients articulate their specific needs and guides them toward potential solutions. The pharmacist might ask, "Would it be helpful for you to be able to monitor your blood pressure at home so you could visit your doctor less often?" The purpose of this step is to ready the patient for a discussion about features and benefits of pharmacy services that meet the stated needs.

- *Step 3: Present features and benefits.* After the patient has identified his or her needs and potential options, the pharmacist presents alternative solutions, concisely describing services and products offered by the pharmacy. If the patient wanted to monitor his blood pressure, the pharmacist might lay out the differences between purchasing home monitoring equipment and using in-store monitoring by the pharmacist or by machine. The information is tailored to the patient's specific needs and preferences.
- *Step 4: Address concerns.* It is common for patients to raise an objection or seek clarification of some issue during the selling process. The key is to listen actively and respond appropriately. Acknowledge the objection, ask further questions, and answer in a way that resolves the objection or negotiates an alternative solution.
- *Step 5: Make the offer.* Once the benefits of a solution have been communicated and all of the objections have been resolved, the pharmacist tries to close the deal by getting a commitment from the patient to act. The action may be to make a purchase, sign a contract to participate in a program, or agree to follow a therapeutic plan.

Personal selling is typically one of the most expensive but most effective forms of promotional communication. It requires the use of highly trained personnel to reach a limited number of customers. It is effective because messages can be individualized to the needs of each customer. Service employees who are able to promote a positive image of a firm can be more valuable than any advertising or sales campaign. Pharmacists can increase their ability to personally sell their ideas by cultivating their credibility and tailoring their messages to the consumer.[18,19]

One widely used personal selling technique is the *elevator speech*—a short, scripted discourse to deliver a message in the time it takes to ride an elevator. This technique involves memorizing and practicing a message that powerfully conveys your ideas in a few words. A good elevator speech can be used to communicate an idea whenever an audience is available for a short time. The marketer can use the elevator speech to take advantage of chance encounters in public settings, at social events, or anywhere people meet.

In social interactions, one of the first questions people ask is "What do you do for a living?" If you reply, "I'm a pharmacist," the other party may respond with a stereotypical comment about pharmacists. However, if your reply is, "I'm a pharmacist who works with patients to control their medical conditions. I have a clinic at Smith's Pharmacy. Here is my card; if you or your friends want to talk about a drug or health issue, call this number and ask for me," you can generate interest in your work, control how people see you, and present a positive image of the profession.

Direct Marketing

Direct marketing is individualized, nonpersonal communication.[3] It is individualized because it targets individual consumers, and it is nonpersonal because consumer contacts come from a database. Database marketing, direct mail, mail order, interactive technology, and computerized telemarketing are other terms used for this type of promotional communication.

The primary components of direct marketing are a customer database and a delivery medium (Figure 11-5). The database contains demographic information, purchasing habits, credit history, behavioral characteristics, and other information collected from a variety of sources, including Web sites, customer surveys, and loyalty card use. The more information the database contains, the more useful it is for identifying and targeting customers. The delivery vehicle is the medium used to contact database customers with a message or offer. Targeted customers might receive discount coupons, free samples, free or discounted services, or reminder messages.

Overuse and misuse of direct marketing has added to negative feelings toward the marketing profession. Most complaints about marketers relate to the intrusive nature of direct marketing; they tend to focus on direct mail, telephone solicitation, or Internet spam. Consumers have learned to cope by using telephone answering machines to screen their calls, throwing away junk mail unopened, and installing software to screen for unsolicited e-mail. In addition, state and federal laws have been passed to regulate direct marketers. The federal Health Insurance Portability and Accountability Act regulates how consumer health data can be collected and used. The Federal Trade Commission's National Do Not Call Registry allows consumers to bar telemarketers from calling them.

FIGURE 11-5 Sources of customer data and examples of media used to deliver direct marketing messages.

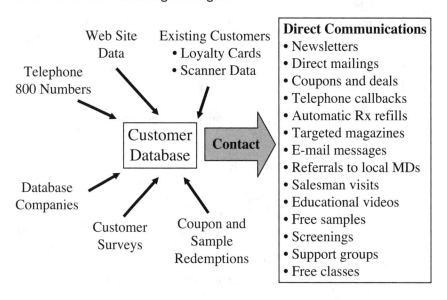

Trust is a key requirement in direct marketing because of the personal nature of much of the information in customer databases. Consumers who think the information is misused can turn from loyal customers into passionate enemies.

Even the appearance of misuse of information can lead to problems. In one exceptional situation, the CVS chain and Giant Pharmacy (associated with the Giant Food grocery chain) received negative publicity in the Washington, D.C., area in 1998 for direct marketing campaigns.[20] The chains sent patient prescription information to a database marketing firm. The database company mailed refill reminders and information about new drugs to database patients. Some patients were upset when they received mailings based on their personal prescription information. When it was learned that drug companies paid the chains and database marketer for the mailings, negative newspaper articles about the practice began appearing. Although the chains argued that they did nothing unethical because the drug companies had no direct access to patient information, public opinion caused CVS and Giant to cancel the mailings.

The following guidelines will help marketers maintain customers' trust as they undertake direct marketing programs:[20]

- All personnel who handle patient data should be trained to do so. Many mistakes can be made by persons who mean well but lack knowledge.
- Consumers should be informed about how their personal data will be used and asked for permission to use the information under specified conditions.
- Consumers should have the ability to opt out of any program. This should be stated up front, so that they do not feel pressured to participate.
- Marketers should fully disclose any conflicts of interest they have. For example, a pharmacist who asks a physician to switch drug brands should explain any financial arrangements through which he or his employer might benefit from the switch.
- Any direct marketing program should be seen as providing good value for all people involved. For those who participate, and even for those who are contacted to participate, the program should offer a clear and obvious advantage. The advantage might be in cost savings or improvements in health. If only the marketer appears to benefit, then consumers lose trust.
- Marketers should take special care with information relating to sensitive medical conditions. For patients with conditions such as AIDS or mental illnesses, release of data can cause tremendous harm.

Sales Promotion

Sales promotion is any promotional communication used to promote a quick sale or action.[3] Examples include price deals, consumer coupons, contests and sweepstakes, refunds and rebates, premium offers, trade promotions, point-of-purchase displays at checkouts, in-store demonstrations, shows and exhibitions, stamps, and sample distribution.

Sales promotion is used to achieve short-term marketing objectives. It promotes immediate behavior, such as purchase of a product or participation in a service. Pharmacies use sales promotion to encourage the sale of merchandise and services. They may have senior citizen days, when all seniors receive a discount on purchases. Using coupons in weekly newspaper advertisements and mailed circulars is also common. Pharmacists frequently waive fees for certain services to reward loyal customers, or offer free initial consultations that encourage patients to sample clinical services. Although pharmacists may not recognize these fee waivers as sales promotion, they are, in effect, a price discount for services.

Sales promotions can be aimed at either consumers or businesses. Those aimed at businesses are called *trade promotions*. They are used by manufacturers and others to encourage retail businesses to put extra effort into promoting certain targeted products. A manufacturer of a non-prescription medication or other product might offer a cash rebate if a certain sales volume of the product is achieved.

One common trade promotion practice is cooperative advertising, in which a manufacturer pays a pharmacy for advertising the manufacturer's product. Another trade promotion practice is paying a pharmacy for filling a certain percentage of prescriptions with generic products or switching from one prescription product to another equally effective product. Pharmacy benefit managers (PBMs) have experimented with using trade promotions to pharmacists, but their efforts have been hindered by state laws that limit rebates (or kickbacks) associated with the dispensing of prescription drugs. Instead, PBMs often write into pharmacy network contracts incentives or penalties that encourage pharmacies to move market share for certain products. Although this may not be labeled as sales promotion, it clearly meets the definition. Many pharmacists resist trade promotions to change therapies because they intrude on the pharmacist–patient relationship.

Sales promotions are best conducted in combination with other forms of marketing communication. A sweepstakes requires advertising to inform consumers about its availability and rules. Coupons often accompany print advertising.

Sales promotions have several strengths compared with other forms of marketing communications. Discounts add value to purchases and induce customers to buy now rather than later. Sales promotions have immediate effects; instead of waiting months to see the impact of an advertising campaign, businesses can evaluate the impact of sales promotions immediately. Sales promotions can also generate excitement about a product. Sales contests, for example, can get people more involved with products than can advertising or other forms of promotion. Sales promotions can induce people to do things they might not ordinarily do, such as put promotional bumper stickers on their cars or engage in crazy stunts to win cash prizes.

Nevertheless, the weaknesses of sales promotions can sometimes outweigh their usefulness. The following weaknesses are associated with sales promotions:[21]

- The benefits of sales promotions are often temporary, with little long-term effect on behavior. Thus, a coupon may get patients to switch pharmacies but do nothing to promote customer loyalty.
- If sales promotions are overused, they can cheapen a brand by over-emphasizing price and minimizing perceptions of quality.

- Sales promotions can hurt pharmacist–patient relationships. Frequent use of discounts could tempt longtime patients to bounce from pharmacy to pharmacy.
- Sales promotions can attract the least profitable customers. Pharmacy sales promotions are likely to attract patients who are more interested in getting discounts than in maintaining a long-term relationship with their pharmacist. These customers are often more costly than loyal customers.
- Discounts from sales promotions can be very expensive. Waiving patient co-payments or offering $10 off for switching a prescription can take a large bite out of a pharmacy's profits.
- Sales promotions can be perceived as manipulative. They reward customers for jumping through hoops. This can irritate customers and is a major reason that some stores offer everyday low prices and minimize sales promotions.

Marketer-Influenced Methods

Public relations and word-of-mouth marketing (commonly called "PR" and "WOM," respectively) are forms of promotion that are influenced, but not controlled, by marketers. Public relations is defined as the process of building a positive image in the minds of the public.[22] It is used to create a supportive climate in the community for your marketing initiatives. Word-of-mouth ("buzz") marketing stimulates discussion of products and services by potential customers.[23–25] While public relations promotes positive images, buzz marketing promotes positive conversation.

Public relations and buzz marketing are third-party techniques; they exert influence indirectly, through parties that are considered to be independent of marketers because they have no clear financial interest in the message. Third-party communications are perceived as more neutral and unbiased than paid forms of promotion such as advertising. This perception can increase attention to and acceptance of the message.

The major advantage of third-party communications—the independence of the communicators—is also a disadvantage. Third parties have no vested interest in conveying the message in the way the marketer desires, and they may distort, ignore, or contest the message. Negative images can be generated just as easily as positive ones. In fact, unfavorable news is likely to spread faster than good news.

Public Relations

Public relations encompasses a broad range of activities to build goodwill and a favorable image of a product or service in the eyes of the public.[22] Pharmacy's "publics," or stakeholders, range from the press to patients to funding agencies.

In the past, public relations was defined by marketers as any nonpaid attempt to get favorable coverage by the news media or to prevent negative coverage.[3] Now, that definition is considered to describe a subset of public relations—publicity. The definition of public relations has been expanded to activities that include[22]

- Lobbying—advocating for a cause with legislatures and government agencies,
- Government relations—communicating with and educating legislatures and government agencies,
- Media relations—dealing with the media to seek publicity or stimulate interest in a cause,
- Publicity—communicating with the public through media (e.g., press releases, news conferences),
- Direct communications with constituents,
- Public appearances before groups (e.g., speeches, seminars), and
- Community relations—dealing with citizens and groups within an area.

Public relations promotes goodwill between marketers and the public. Goodwill toward the pharmacy profession is formed from positive images of and mental associations with pharmacists, pharmacy employees, and pharmacies. Public relations attempts to build positive images where they are absent, strengthen existing positive images, and repair any negative images that exist. The stronger and more positive the image communicated, the greater are the goodwill and consequent support for a cause.

Publicity is a key element of public relations. Pharmacists use publicity extensively to influence media coverage of the profession. Media coverage can be generated by

- Speaking to a community group about nonprescription medications,
- Participating in an "adopt-a-highway" program,
- Sponsoring a baseball team,
- Lobbying to expand the role of pharmacists,
- Demonstrating a new flavoring system to make drugs more acceptable to pediatric patients,
- Holding poison prevention programs,
- Sending National Pharmacy Week press releases,
- Offering free blood pressure screenings,
- Sponsoring public service announcements, and
- Writing letters to the editor about negative depiction of a pharmacist in the news.

Publicity events may cost money, but they are less expensive than advertising and other forms of promotional communication. The primary cost results from the time and effort spent managing the message (which can be considerable).

The negative side of promotion through publicity is that, once in the hands of the media, the message can be ignored, de-emphasized, or distorted. Indeed, a television reporter can turn a pharmacist interview originally focused on how pharmacists reduce medication errors into a story about how pharmacists are not doing enough to reduce errors.

Word-of-Mouth Marketing

Word-of-mouth or buzz marketing encourages unpaid but influential individuals to generate conversation about ideas, products, or services. Buzz has a connection to public relations; just as good public relations can cause buzz, buzz can cause good public relations. The primary difference is that buzz marketing focuses on promoting in-person discussion, while public relations emphasizes the development of goodwill.

Buzz spreads when extraordinary things are talked about. When people are exposed to a noteworthy idea or object, they want to tell others. The more remarkable or "sticky" the topic, the more likely it is to generate buzz. The value of buzz lies in its ability to encourage people to try new products, adopt fresh ideas, and use innovations.

Pharmacists can best promote buzz about their products and services as part of an integrated communication strategy, incorporating advertising and other techniques that reinforce and support each other. Table 11-2[25] provides steps in a buzz marketing strategy.

Like public relations, buzz marketing has downsides. Buzz can be negative as well as positive. It turns negative if it stimulates demand that outstrips supply and customers become frustrated. Furthermore, buzz marketing can backfire if it leads consumers to feel deceived or manipulated by marketers. Some buzz marketing firms have misrepresented paid

TABLE 11-2   Steps in Spreading Buzz

Choose a buzz-worthy idea	A buzz-worthy idea must be innovative, personally relevant, and clearly superior to what is currently available. Visible and tangible objects are more likely to generate conversation. An interesting story will make the idea more likely to be recalled and shared with others. A life-saving drug discovered in an Amazon rain forest or at the bottom of an ocean will generate buzz better than a new drug insurance plan.

TABLE 11-2   Steps in Spreading Buzz (*continued*)

Identify opinion leaders among the group you wish to influence.	Opinion leaders have greater influence on the spread of ideas because they are "connected"; they readily interact with others by nature or through their work. They are up-to-date with new trends and freely express their views. They may feel and act differently from others and be more likely to rebel against the status quo.
Approach opinion leaders in a way that gets them talking.	People talk about the extraordinary, not the commonplace. Thus, buzz is driven by the marketer's imagination; a quirky advertisement or outrageous promotional stunt can help spread buzz about a product. Controversy can generate buzz, and so can extremes (e.g., top 10 or worst 5 lists). Some marketers generate buzz by promoting the existence of a "secret" and making people guess what it is. Sometimes an object or idea itself is sufficient to get people talking, particularly if the marketer provides samples or a demonstration.
Identify and overcome obstacles and bottlenecks to adoption.	Buzz can be stopped at any time in its early development. Negative word-of-mouth caused by an unmet expectation or bad experience can halt buzz in its tracks. Marketers must continually assess peoples' experience with innovations to determine the degree to which they meet expectations and needs. Problems with the product itself should be resolved immediately. Any systemic barriers that could hamper adoption should be identified and addressed.
Use different channels of communication.	Buzz marketing is typically integrated with other promotional communications. Combining buzz with other methods can broaden the reach and effectiveness of promotional messages.
Encourage adaptation.	If an innovation is not used exactly as it was originally designed, that is OK. Adaptation of innovations to new situations is common; it should be encouraged because it helps facilitate adoption. Adaptation works best when individuals use innovations to resolve their own needs, and not necessarily the needs intended by marketers.
Ask for an endorsement.	Once opinion leaders have adopted an innovation, get their endorsement. Have them comment on the innovation, and get permission to quote them in promotional fliers and advertisements. Encourage them to tell others about the benefits of the innovation. If they willingly champion the innovation, get permission to refer others to them to hear about their experience.

Source: Reference 25.

marketing as spontaneous word-of-mouth; they have paid "shoppers" to visit Web sites or trendy locations and rave about products. Buzz marketers have also paid for ghost-written promotional pieces and represented them as unbiased work.

Deceptive buzz tactics can destroy the credibility of marketing messages and make consumers even more cynical and suspicious toward marketers. Pharmacists should use buzz sparingly and cautiously. A poorly planned and initiated campaign can damage consumers' confidence in pharmacists and the perception of pharmacists as credible advocates for patients.

DEVELOPING A PROMOTIONAL PLAN

A promotional plan is an outline for accomplishing marketing objectives. It is an element of the overall marketing plan. It requires a clear understanding of the product, customers, competitors, price, and target market. A promotional plan typically consists of the following steps:

1. Defining the objective of the promotion,
2. Crafting a message and a strategy for delivering it,
3. Selecting an integrated communication mix, and
4. Measuring the effectiveness of the promotion.

Defining the Objective

Promotional objectives should originate from and complement the overall objectives established in the marketing plan, so that communications will supplement and reinforce other elements of the marketing mix. Accordingly, if a pharmacist's professional image is a major part of the overall plan, then pricing, communications, pharmacy location, and all other elements of the marketing mix should reinforce this image of professionalism.

Promotional objectives are usually based on a statement about the positioning strategy for the business or product. This positioning strategy statement defines the product or services provided, target consumer, market, competition, and meaningful features of the product or business that differentiate it from competitors. The positioning statement may also describe the personality of the brand, which will be established and reinforced in all promotional communications. The following is an example of a positioning statement that might be written for a community pharmacy:

Johnson's Apothecary provides professional pharmacist services, pharmacy products, and merchandise to consumers on the north side of the city and commuters in the northern suburbs. Johnson's Apothecary is a locally owned, family-run organization that takes care of people, not medical conditions. The owner and other pharmacists are well known and respected in the community. Two pharmacists are certified diabetes educators. The merchandise selection emphasizes health care over general merchandise. Personal service is paramount. Johnson's is also a meeting place for locals who just want to chat.

All marketing communications should bolster the image promoted in the positioning statement. Sales promotions, advertising, and public relations events should be crafted with an eye toward their contribution to a consistent image. This will help ensure that the same message is repeated in multiple ways and media.

The desired outcome of promoting pharmacy products and pharmacist services might be to inform, persuade, or remind:

- Inform
  - Inform people about new products or services.
  - Increase awareness or comprehension of services.
  - Educate people about their medications.
- Persuade
  - Persuade people to buy.
  - Persuade people of the value of a product or service.
  - Enhance and reinforce the image of pharmacists.
  - Emphasize an advantage of one product over another.
- Remind
  - Remind people about the availability of services and products.
  - Remind people to seek care for medical conditions.

It is clear from these examples that increasing sales is not the immediate goal of all marketing communication. In many cases, the priority might be to influence a person's attitude toward or knowledge about pharmaceutical services or products. Nevertheless, it is important to remember that the ultimate goal is to influence some action by the consumer. Changing attitudes and knowledge is important only if it leads eventually to some action desired by the marketer, such as making a purchase or being compliant with drug therapy.

Crafting a Message and Strategy

This step in the promotional plan involves deciding what one wants to say to target customers and determining how to say it. A pharmacist may wish to promote the message that pharmaceutical care is beneficial to patients. The pharmacist then needs to list a number of benefits that can be highlighted for consumers: Pharmaceutical care helps people take control of their health; saves people money; helps people understand their medications and make better decisions about them; helps people live happier, healthier lives; and saves lives.

The pharmacist can then design a message that will capture these benefits in a way that will be meaningful to customers. This is easier said than done. The pharmacist must choose a benefit that appeals to the target customers, compose a message that will capture the mind of the consumer, and deliver it in a way that will encourage action. It is best to keep the message simple.

Formulating a message to consumers requires the marketer to solve four problems:[26]

1. *What to say (message content):* How will the message appeal to the receiver's self-interest, emotions, or moral viewpoints?
2. *How to say it in words (message structure):* Will the message be even-handed or biased? How will the message be organized?
3. *How to say it in images (message format):* What images or pictures will be used to get the message across? The answer depends on the medium used to communicate the message.
4. *Who should say it (message source):* Messages delivered by attractive sources achieve higher levels of attention and recall. The expertise, trustworthiness, and likability of the source delivering the message are all important.

The message should revolve around some unique selling proposition[7] —or "big idea." A unique selling proposition communicates information about product features and benefits that are meaningful to target consumers. Selling propositions are based on the positioning strategy. A unique selling proposition for a pharmacy might be, "All of our pharmacists are certified diabetes educators who will help you with your diabetes care needs."

Selecting a Communication Mix

Usually, an integrated mix of promotional methods is used to communicate a message to consumers. The use of multiple methods increases the number of opportunities for new and existing customers to receive a message. Not all people read the newspaper, listen to the radio, are connected to the Internet, and watch television, but most people take part in at least one of these activities. A message can be reinforced by communicating it in different ways. A television advertisement can increase awareness of pharmacy services, a coupon can get a consumer to visit a pharmacy, and a pharmacist can personally sell the value of pharmaceutical care.

The selection of media depends on the budget for promotional communications and which promotional media will be most efficient and effective in influencing target customers. A rule of thumb is that the cost increases as more people are reached with the marketing message and as the message is more personalized.

Promotions on the Internet seem to break this rule, since it is possible to send a message on the Web to millions of people for very little money. A promotional message in a blog, video clip, or e-mail can spread like a virus through professional and social Web networks; this is an inexpensive means of making an exponential impact on thoughts and behaviors. The right message at the right time in the right way can spread rapidly across the world.

Measuring the Result

In designing promotional plans, it is important to define success by some objective measure. There is no way to know if promotional communications are successful until their results are measured. Ways to measure the success of marketing communications include the following:

- Examining changes in sales after promotional events,
- Asking new customers how they heard about your business,
- Asking patients if they remember seeing your mailed brochure and if they can describe what it said, and
- Observing whether consumer behavior changes; for example, did a patient who was enrolled in a smoking cessation program stop smoking?

SUMMARY

All pharmacists engage in marketing communication. Some do so better than others. Understanding the communication model and the information processing model can help pharmacists craft effective communications and avoid common blunders.

Advertising, public relations, personal selling, direct marketing, and sales promotion are used to promote marketing messages. The form of promotion used depends on the objective of the communication, the message itself, and the cost of delivering it. The most important measure of any marketing communication is whether it results in some desired behavior by the targeted receiver.

References

1. Higgins D. *The Art of Writing Advertising: Conversations with Masters of the Craft.* Lincolnwood, Ill: NTC Business Books; 1990:93.
2. Fleming H Jr. The new spinners. *Drug Top.* June 1, 1998,142:50–4.
3. Kotler P. *Marketing Management: Analysis, Planning, and Control.* 4th ed. Englewood Cliffs, NJ: Prentice Hall; 1980.
4. Dickinson JG. Is pharmacy heading for a fall? *US Pharm.* July 1997;12: 37–8.
5. Hasegawa GR. The image of pharmacy. *Am J Health Syst Pharm.* 1996;53: 1541.
6. Posey LM. Image problem in clinical pharmacy. *Consult Pharm.* 1987;2: 265.
7. Schultz DE, Tannenbaum SI, Lauterborn RF. *The New Marketing Paradigm.* Lincolnwood, Ill: NTC Business Books; 1993.
8. Engel JF, Blackwell RD, Miniard PW. *Consumer Behavior.* Fort Worth, Tex: Dryden Press; 1993.
9. Smith W. Evidence for the effectiveness of techniques to change physician behavior. *Chest.* 2000;118(2):8S–17S.
10. Soumerai SB, Avorn J. Principles of educational outreach ('academic detailing') to improve clinical decision making. *JAMA.* 1990;263:549–56.
11. Burton B, Rowell A. Unhealthy spin. *BMJ.* 2003; 26(7400):1205.
12. Berry LL. On great service: a framework for action. *J Mark.* 1998;62:123–5.
13. Hill CJ, Gandhi N. Service advertising: a framework to its effectiveness. *J Serv Mark.* 1992;6(4):63–76.
14. Zeithaml VA, Parasuraman A, Berry LL. Problems and strategies in services marketing. *J Mark.* Spring 1985;49:33–46.
15. Holdford DA, Yom SH. Content analysis of newspaper advertising of pharmacy services. *J Pharm Mark Manage.* 2003;15(2):81–96.
16. Jolles RL. *Customer Centered Selling.* New York: Simon and Schuster; 1998.
17. McDonough RP, Doucette WR. Using personal selling skills to promote pharmacy services. *J Am Pharm Assoc.* 2003;43:363–72.
18. Holdford DA. Marketing your ideas through persuasion. *APhA Career Manager.* Summer 1999:1–8.
19. Conger JA. The necessary art of persuasion. *Harv Bus Rev.* 1998;76(3): 84–97.
20. Lo B, Alpers A. Uses and abuses of prescription drug information in pharmacy benefits management programs. *JAMA.* 2000;283:801–6.
21. Bradley F. *Marketing Management: Providing, Communicating and Delivering Value.* Upper Saddle River, NJ: Prentice Hall; 1995.
22. Pugliese TL. *Public Relations for Pharmacists.* Washington, DC: American Pharmaceutical Association; 2000.
23. Rosen E. *The Anatomy of Buzz: How to Create Word-of-Mouth Marketing.* New York: Doubleday; 2002.
24. Dye R. The buzz on buzz. *Harv Bus Rev.* 2000;78(6):139–46.
25. Holdford DA. Using buzz to promote ideas, services, and products. *J Am Pharm Assoc.* 2004;44:387–96.
26. Wells W, Burnett J, Moriarty S. *Advertising: Principles and Practice.* Englewood Cliffs, NJ: Prentice Hall; 1992.

Additional Readings

Berry LL. Big ideas in services marketing. *J Serv Mark.* 1987;3(2):5–9.

Berwick DM. Disseminating innovations in health care. *JAMA.* 2003;289: 1969–75.

Cialdini RB. *Influence: The Psychology of Persuasion.* New York: William Morrow and Co Inc; 1993.

Clancy KJ, Shulman RS. *The Marketing Revolution: A Radical Manifesto for Dominating the Marketplace.* New York: Harper Business; 1991.

Gladwell M. *The Tipping Point.* New York: Time Warner; 2000.

Levinson JC. *Guerrilla Marketing: Secrets for Making Big Profits from Your Small Business.* Boston: Houghton Mifflin; 1984.

Silverman G. *The Secrets of Word-of-Mouth Marketing: How to Trigger Exponential Sales Through Runaway Word of Mouth.* New York: American Management Association Books; 2001.

Exercises and Questions

1. Use the communication model in Figure 11-2 to describe why it is so hard for marketers to get their messages to consumers.
2. Use the information processing model to compare the relative effectiveness of a newspaper pharmacy advertisement, a television advertisement, and personal selling by a pharmacist in getting a patient to take some action.
3. What are important things to consider when designing a promotional communication?
4. Discuss factors that go into a pharmacy's choice of a promotional medium.
5. Why might selling patient data to drug companies for direct marketing hurt the image of pharmacists?
6. Debate the value and costs of drug company rebates to pharmacists for switching drug brands.

Activities

1. Look at a pharmacy advertisement in your local newspaper (hint: Sunday papers frequently have pharmacy advertising inserts) or on an Internet Web site. How much of the total ad content is devoted to nondrug merchandise, nonprescription medicines, and prescription medicines and services? Describe the image of prescription drugs and services presented in the advertisement. Would you say that the ad enhances, detracts from, or has little impact on the image of pharmacists? Why?
2. Using information from the section "Developing a promotional plan" (pages 258 to 261), create a promotional plan for your program or service. Be sure to include a position statement that describes the service, your target patients, the market, competition, and meaningful benefits of the service.

PART VI

PRICING AND PLACING PHARMACIST SERVICES

CHAPTER 12

PRICING PHARMACIST SERVICES

By Norman V. Carroll, PhD

Professor of Pharmacy Administration
Virginia Commonwealth University School of Pharmacy

Objectives

After studying this chapter, the reader should be able to

❑ Explain why pricing is an important part of marketing pharmacy products and services.
❑ Discuss how pricing relates to other elements of the marketing mix.
❑ List and discuss the effects of consumer-related factors, competition, pharmacy objectives, and costs on pricing decisions.
❑ Calculate the cost of providing a pharmacist service.
❑ Explain the relationships among price, cost, and demand for a pharmacist service.
❑ List and explain the steps involved in one strategy for pricing pharmacist services.
❑ List and explain methods of presenting service prices to consumers.

Old City Pharmacy is planning to start a smoking cessation clinic for its patients. The service will provide patients with nicotine gum and behavioral counseling to help them stop smoking. The pharmacy manager estimates that each course of treatment will require an 8-week supply of nicotine gum and about 5 hours of counseling over the course of 12 weeks. The costs of providing the service will include the pharmacist's salary, renovation of the pharmacy to provide a private counseling area, training for the pharmacist, promotion of the service, and the cost of the nicotine gum. A major concern is how to price the service.

The price of a pharmacist service—such as smoking cessation assistance—is the amount of money the pharmacy asks a patient to give up in order to buy the service. This is a value-based transaction. The patient will purchase the service only if he or she believes that its value exceeds its price. Whether the patient believes this depends on a number of factors:

> *The optimal price for a service is the price that is less than its perceived value to consumers and greater than the pharmacy's cost of providing it.*

- The consumer's perceived need for the service,
- How well the service is provided,
- How convenient it is for the patient to get the service,
- How well the benefits of the service are explained,
- Whether the patient believes the pharmacist is the appropriate person to provide the service, and
- The availability of other providers of the service (i.e., competitors).

In other words, the consumer's assessment of the value of a service depends not only on price, but on all elements of the marketing mix. This has several important implications for setting prices. First, managers should carefully consider the service's value to the consumer. The pharmacist may think that the service provides value to the consumer, and the service may actually do so, but unless the consumer believes the service has value he or she will not be willing to pay for it. Second, the price selected must be consistent with other elements of the marketing mix. The service itself and the manner in which it is provided, promoted, and delivered must convey the same message about the service's value as the price does. Third, cost is not the only, or even the primary, factor in determining the appropriate price. Consumers' perceptions of the service and of the competition are at least as important. The optimal price for a service is the price that is less than its perceived value to consumers and greater than the pharmacy's cost of providing it.

If the pharmacy used a cost-based approach to pricing, it would first estimate the costs of providing the service, then set a price to cover those costs plus profit. This approach fails to consider the value of the service to consumers. If consumers do not believe the price reflects good value, they will not buy the service.

A more rational approach, and one that is more consistent with a marketing philosophy, is to first consider the value that the service provides to the consumer, next set a price that reflects the service's value, and then determine how to provide the service at a cost that makes this

TABLE 12-1   Factors Affecting Price

Consumer-related factors
  Demand
  Pharmacy image
  Price as a signal of quality
  Nonmonetary costs
  Set price offered to pharmacy
Competition
Pharmacy objectives
  Maximizing long-term profits
  Penetration
  Skimming
  Maintaining the status quo
Costs
  Service costs
  Material and supply costs
  Net profit

price profitable. Although this approach is less intuitive than a cost-based approach, it recognizes the primacy of the consumer in making pricing decisions. Factors that managers need to consider when setting prices (Table 12-1) are discussed in this chapter.

CONSUMER-RELATED FACTORS AFFECTING PRICES

Value must be determined from the consumer's point of view. Consumer-related factors affecting price include demand, pharmacy image, price as a signal of quality, nonmonetary costs, and, when third-party payers set prices, determining how the service can be provided profitably.

Demand

The primary consumer-related factor that managers must consider is demand. Demand refers to the quantity of a product or service that consumers will buy at a given price. Demand is related to, but different from, need. The need for pharmacy products and pharmacist services can be objectively determined by medical experts on the basis of prevalence of disease in the population. Demand, on the other hand, is based on consumer perceptions. A pharmacy that serves a large population of smokers can reasonably assume that there is a large need for smoking cessation services. However, if the patients have no desire to quit smoking, or if they

believe that pharmacist-provided
services are of no value in helping
them quit, then there is little demand
for the service.

> *Price elasticity of demand is a measure of how sensitive consumers are to different price levels.*

Because demand is based on consumer perceptions, it can be affected
by marketing activities. Skillful advertising and promotion can increase
demand for a product or service. As a result of heavy, skillful promotion,
there is a substantial demand for cigarettes, even though there is no need
for the product.

Demand is also affected by price. As the price of a product or service
rises, the quantity demanded by consumers usually falls. The extent to
which the quantity demanded changes in response to price is known as
the *price elasticity of demand*. It is a measure of how sensitive consumers
are to different price levels. Different products and services have different
levels of elasticity or price sensitivity. Knowing how sensitive consumers
are to prices for a service—that is, knowing the demand for a service—is
critical to setting an appropriate price.

Figure 12-1 illustrates different price elasticities of demand. One curve
illustrates the price elasticity of a product with elastic demand. Notice
that a change in price from $40 to $20 leads to a disproportionately greater

FIGURE 12-1   Elastic and inelastic demand.

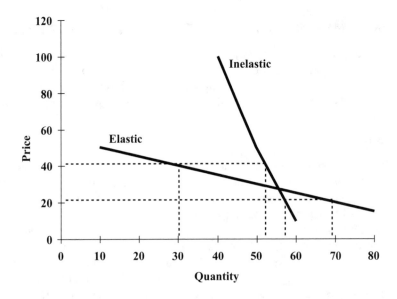

change in the quantity demanded—from 30 units to 69 units. Elastic demand means that consumers are very sensitive to price differences. The second curve in the figure illustrates inelastic demand. Here, a change in price from $40 to $20 leads to a smaller increase in quantity—from 52 to 58 units. Inelastic demand means consumers are much less sensitive to price differences.

Dolan[1] and Nagle and Holden[2] suggest that managers use the following guidelines to estimate consumers' price sensitivity for a specific product or service.

1. The consumer's sensitivity to price increases as the price of the product or service becomes a greater part of the total cost of therapy. The total cost of treating coughs and colds is low, so consumers are quite sensitive to the price of pharmacist counseling for cough and cold products. A high price for this service will probably result in little or no demand. The total treatment costs of asthma, on the other hand, are quite high. They include expensive drug therapy, frequent physician monitoring, trips to the emergency room, and hospitalizations. Compared with the total costs of treating asthma, the costs of asthma-related counseling provided by pharmacists are small. Therefore, consumers are likely to be less sensitive to the price of asthma counseling services.
2. Consumers' sensitivity to price is higher when there are minimal differences among competing products and services. Further, price sensitivity increases as consumers find it easier to compare products and services. This depends on how competent consumers are to judge differences in quality and how convenient it is for them to do so. Nonprescription drugs, for example, are standardized products. Consumers get the same product whether they buy it at a supermarket, a discount store, or an apothecary shop. Assuming there are no meaningful differences in the services that accompany the product, consumers can make their choice on the basis of price. Because the products are standardized, it is easy to obtain and compare prices. Thus, price differences can have a major effect on where consumers purchase nonprescription drugs. Pharmacist services, on the other hand, are not standardized. The quality of services provided in different pharmacies and by different pharmacists varies a great deal. This makes it difficult for consumers to compare services. They have to actually receive the services, or observe them being provided, to be able to evaluate them. Further, it is more difficult for consumers to judge the quality of services than of products. Consumers can assess interpersonal aspects of services, but they are usually not able to judge technical merit. Consequently, consumers are less sensitive to the price of services.

3. Consumers' price sensitivity increases as switching costs increase. Switching costs are the costs—both monetary and nonmonetary—that consumers incur when they change their source of supply for a product or service. If a particular pharmacy is much more convenient for consumers, then they will incur significant time costs in switching their purchases to another pharmacy. Because of the time and trouble involved in using another pharmacy, consumers are unlikely to change pharmacies solely because of differences in prescription prices. Services that require a relationship to be built between the consumer and the provider have high switching costs. If a consumer switched lawyers in the middle of a complicated case, the consumer would have to repeat with the new lawyer the process of providing all relevant information about the case, developing rapport, and developing a strategy for the case. Patients who build relationships with pharmacists through receipt of patient-oriented services over a long period of time face similar switching costs.

The manager must have a good estimate of demand for a service before the service can be priced. Considering consumers' price sensitivity aids the manager is estimating demand. For a more in-depth discussion of demand estimation, readers can refer to publications by Nagle and Holden[2], Simon[3], and Carroll.[4]

Pharmacy Image

Initially, consumers choose a pharmacy on the basis of what they perceive the pharmacy's prices and services to be, not necessarily what they actually are. Consumer perceptions are based largely on the pharmacy's image. This is especially true for price. Most consumers choosing a pharmacy are not familiar with the pharmacy's prices or how that pharmacy's prices compare with another's. At best, consumers who take maintenance medications know how much a few pharmacies charge for the medications they buy regularly.

Because consumers are generally unfamiliar with prices, the pharmacy's price image is determined by the pharmacy's overall image, which, in turn, is determined by all the elements of the marketing mix. For example, a small, apothecary-type pharmacy located in a medical center is likely to have a high-service, high-price image. If its pharmacists spend a great deal of time counseling patients and the pharmacy carries only drugs and health care supplies, consumers are even more likely to have this image. On the other hand, a pharmacy located in a mass merchandiser, such as Kmart or Wal-Mart, is likely to be perceived as a low-price, discount pharmacy. This image is reinforced by weekly advertisements for sale-priced nonprescription merchandise and in-store signage announcing the store as the "low-cost leader."

Because image strongly affects consumer perceptions of price, managers need to offer prices that are consistent with the pharmacy's image. The apothecary pharmacy is expected, because of its image, to have higher prices. Even if it actually offers discount prices, few consumers are likely to be aware of the low prices. Most continue to perceive it as a high-price pharmacy, so there is little to be gained by offering discount prices. On the other hand, a pharmacy that appears to be a discount pharmacy but charges high prices has little to offer to consumers who ultimately discover that it does not offer discount prices.

Price as a Signal of Quality

Consumers sometimes use price as an indicator of quality. This is especially likely for services, because consumers have more difficulty judging the quality of services than of products. Services are intangible, less frequently advertised than products, and less likely than products to be associated with brand names. Consumers use both brand names and frequency of advertising as indicators of quality.

Consumers may assume that higher-priced services are of higher quality, particularly when there is great variability in the quality of service provided and when the service is seen as involving high risk to the consumer (e.g., surgery). Many pharmacist services fall into this category; there is likely to be great variability in the quality of services provided, and many—such as counseling and monitoring asthma patients—may be seen as high-risk services. Low prices for such services may actually decrease demand by signaling low quality to consumers.

Nonmonetary Costs

In addition to the prices they pay for pharmacy products and pharmacist services, patients incur time costs for traveling to the pharmacy and waiting for services to be delivered, and search costs in trying to find the products and services they need. They incur psychic costs by worrying about whether their medicines will help or harm them. Zeithaml and Bitner[5] point out that for some patients nonmonetary costs may outweigh monetary costs. Consequently, managers need to carefully consider how the products and services they offer affect nonmonetary costs.

Many pharmacy services strongly affect nonmonetary costs. Delivery services, for example, decrease consumers' time costs. Patient education and counseling initially increase time costs because consumers must

spend time interacting with pharmacists. On the other hand, these services reduce psychic costs and may,
in the long run, reduce time costs. A
few minutes spent discussing medications with the pharmacist may be
more than compensated for by the
time saved by preventing adverse
reactions or treatment failures.

> *The pharmacy's goal in demand backward pricing is not to determine an optimal price for its services, but to determine how it can profitably provide the service at the offered price.*

Set Price Offered

In 2005 third-party payers (such as Medicaid, private insurance plans,
and health maintenance organizations) paid for 87% of prescriptions dispensed by retail pharmacies (including chains, independents, supermarket and discount store pharmacies, and mail order pharmacies).[6] In
almost all cases the third-party payer, not the pharmacy, set the prescription price. As third-party reimbursement for patient care services grows,
pharmacies may find themselves in the same situation in regard to the
pricing of services.

Marketers refer to this situation as *demand backward pricing*. The pharmacy's goal in demand backward pricing is not to determine an optimal
price for its services, but to determine how it can profitably provide the
service at the offered price. Much of the literature and training material on providing patient care services has assumed a demand backward
framework. For example, most programs for helping pharmacists implement patient care services in community pharmacies include substantial
discussion of changing the pharmacy's workflow so that pharmacists
have more time to care for patients. Usually this involves turning more
dispensing-related tasks over to technicians and increasing automation in
the pharmacy. The goal is to allow pharmacies to be able to provide patient
care services without increasing the pharmacy's costs. The assumption
behind this goal is that the reimbursement pharmacies receive will be so
low that they will have to change the way they operate in order to provide
the services profitably.

COMPETITION

A pharmacy must consider the prices charged by the pharmacies and
health care practitioners with which it competes. Unless a pharmacy has
some major advantage over its competitors, such as more convenient location, friendlier personnel, or better services, it will not be able to charge
substantially higher prices. A pharmacy that has a distinct advantage will

be able to charge higher prices only if it can convince consumers of the value of the advantage.

Because most pharmacies do not provide patient care services other than counseling, it may be easy to believe that a pharmacy has no competition for these services. This is not true. Many of these services—such as monitoring warfarin and cholesterol levels, teaching patients to use a glucometer, or counseling about smoking cessation—are also provided by physicians, physician extenders, and nurses. Thus, the prices these providers charge must be considered in setting pharmacy prices.

Consumers frequently have in mind what they believe is a reasonable price to pay for a product or service. This is known as a *reference price.* Consumers' reference price for a can of soda from a vending machine—how much they expect to pay—is probably between 50 cents and $1. Most consumers would not be willing to pay more than that under normal conditions. Reference prices are developed from experience purchasing the same or similar items. Managers should consider reference prices in determining prices of pharmacist services. For example, if a physician's office visit for warfarin monitoring, including laboratory work, costs a consumer $100, that may be the consumer's reference price for a similar service offered in a pharmacy.

PHARMACY OBJECTIVES

A pharmacy's pricing should be consistent with its overall objectives. The objective of most pharmacies is to maximize long-term profits. To do this, the manager must set prices low enough to attract and retain customers and high enough to yield a profit. This strategy allows the pharmacy to make a reasonable profit over many years. Although maximizing long-term profit is the most common objective, other objectives are important in particular situations.

A new pharmacy, or a pharmacy offering a new service, might have the objective of rapidly building sales volume. To meet this objective, the pharmacy would offer low prices to attract business. This strategy sacrifices short-term profits in order to build sales quickly. This is called a *penetration pricing* strategy. It is preferred in situations where demand is highly elastic (i.e., consumers are price sensitive), where there is strong competition, and where increased volume leads to economies of scale.

Some pharmacies use *loss leaders* to increase sales and profits. Loss leaders are typically high-demand products or services for which prices are well known. A loss leader strategy involves selling these products at or below cost in order to attract consumers into the pharmacy. The pharmacy expects these consumers to also buy other, more profitable, goods and services. Loss leader pricing differs from penetration pricing in that the former offers low prices only on a few selected products whereas the latter offers low prices on a wide range of products.

Other pharmacies have the objective of serving only those consumers who are willing to pay higher prices. This is a *price-skimming* strategy. It usually requires offering a service that is not widely available or offering a level of overall service that other pharmacies cannot or choose not to provide. Many specialist physicians and lawyers use a price-skimming strategy; they serve only those consumers who are willing to pay for their higher levels of training and expertise.

Price skimming can also be used to price a new product or service. This is done when the business would like to maximize its profits on the service quickly. Price skimming is most appropriate for pricing new products and services when there are a substantial number of price-insensitive consumers and few substitutes for the service. Pharmaceutical companies that develop therapeutically unique products, especially first products in a new therapeutic class, usually use price skimming when the product is introduced. Businesses that introduce products and services at a skimming price typically lower the price over time. They do this to attract additional business by serving more price-sensitive markets.

A pharmacy may have an objective of maintaining the status quo. This is an appropriate objective for a pharmacy that earns acceptable profits, faces strong competitors, and has no distinct advantage over its competitors. In this situation, a pharmacy might be quite happy to maintain the current situation. This could best be accomplished by pricing at the same level as the competition. Pricing higher would lead to a substantial loss of sales (because the pharmacy would have no advantage to attract consumers), and pricing lower could start a price war with competitors (because they also have no advantage to attract consumers). So, the pharmacy's best strategy is to set its prices to match those of its competitors.

COSTS

The price of a pharmacist service must be sufficient to cover service costs, material and supply costs, and net profit. Service costs include salaries, rent and utilities, depreciation, and insurance required to provide the service. The cost of supplies or materials needed to provide the service will be referred to in this chapter as product costs. Finally, there is profit (also called net income). The service cost is usually the largest component of the cost of providing a service, but there may also be product costs. For example, as part of a pharmacy's smoking cessation service, nicotine gum may be used to help patients quit smoking.

If a pharmacy is to earn a satisfactory profit, its prices must cover its costs plus some surplus for net income. This is more complicated than it may seem, because costs, sales volume, and price are interrelated. Changes in one usually result in changes in the others.

Calculating Service Costs

The service cost is the average, or per unit, cost of providing the service. Service costs include the expenses directly incurred in providing the product or service and a fair share of expenses incurred indirectly. To accurately calculate service costs, a manager must understand several different kinds of costs, including fixed and variable costs and direct and indirect costs, and how they are related.

Fixed and Variable Costs

The total costs of providing a service can be broken into fixed and variable costs. *Fixed costs* are those that remain the same regardless of volume. Depreciation is a fixed cost. No matter how high the pharmacy's sales go during a given year, the depreciation expense will not change. This is because depreciation is based on the value of fixed assets, which is not directly affected by changes in sales. Other examples of fixed costs include property taxes, managers' salaries, and business licenses.

Services frequently have high fixed costs. A community pharmacy might hire a new pharmacist specifically to implement a warfarin monitoring service and agree to pay her $80,000 per year regardless of the volume of warfarin monitoring services provided. In this case, the pharmacist's salary would be a fixed cost.

Fixed costs can be plotted as shown in Figure 12-2. The figure indicates that fixed costs of providing a smoking cessation service are $28,000.

Variable costs increase in direct proportion to increases in volume. Sometimes the provision of services is structured to include significant variable costs. For example, assume that a pharmacy is implementing a smoking cessation clinic. The manager is not sure what volume of services will be demanded, so he is reluctant to add another pharmacist. Instead, he agrees to pay one of the current pharmacists to work additional hours to operate the smoking cessation service. In this situation, as the volume of services provided increases, so does the number of hours the pharmacist works. Since the service-related salary expense grows in direct proportion to increases in the volume of smoking cessation service provided, salary expense for the service is a variable cost. Variable costs for the smoking cessation service are $0 when no patients are served and rise to $20,000

FIGURE 12-2 Costs of providing smoking cessation services.

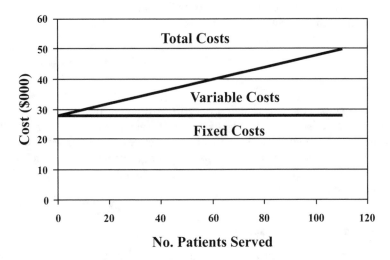

when 100 patients are served. Since total costs are the sum of fixed and variable costs, in Figure 12-2 total costs are $28,000 when no patients are served and $48,000 when 100 patients are served.

Direct and Indirect Costs

Another way of categorizing costs is as direct and indirect. *Direct costs* are those that are directly caused by or result from providing the service. Direct costs of providing a smoking cessation service include pharmacists' time spent counseling and educating patients, patient education materials, and the cost of any products (such as nicotine gum) used to assist patients in quitting. Direct costs may also be thought of as those costs that the pharmacy would not incur if it did not provide the service. If the pharmacy did not dispense prescriptions, it would not incur the costs of prescription containers or pharmacy licenses.

Indirect costs are those that are not directly caused by or do not directly result from providing the service. They are costs that the pharmacy would incur even if it did not provide the service in question. Examples include rent, utilities, and the manager's salary. These costs are shared costs or joint costs, in the sense that they are necessary for the sale of all the pharmacy's products and services. If the pharmacy did not provide smoking cessation services, it would continue to incur indirect costs.

The previous paragraph describes indirect costs as defined in accounting, but in health economics the definition is different. There, indirect costs are the value of lost productivity that patients and society incur as a result of mortality or morbidity. A carpenter who contracts AIDS may no longer be able to work. The value of the work he is no longer able to do is considered an indirect cost of the illness. Similarly, patients may not be able to work while experiencing migraine headaches; the value of the work they are not able to do during a headache is an indirect cost of migraine.

The cost of providing a particular service includes all direct costs and a fair share of indirect costs. A basic problem in calculating a service cost is determining what is a fair share. For example, how much of the rent should be recognized as part of the cost of the smoking cessation service and how much should be recognized as an expense of the rest of the pharmacy? Determining how much of an indirect cost should be recognized, or assigned to, a particular service is a problem of *allocating costs*. A full discussion of pharmacy-related cost allocation can be found in reference 7.

Example: Costs of Providing a Smoking Cessation Service

This chapter began with the question of how to price a smoking cessation service provided in a community pharmacy. A major consideration in setting a price is estimating the average, or per unit, cost of providing the service. Estimating the average cost of providing smoking cessation services to a patient is complicated by the interdependency of price, demand, and cost.

The manager of Old City Pharmacy believes that the smoking cessation service will incur the following costs (Table 12-2):

TABLE 12-2   Estimated Annual Costs ($) of Smoking Cessation Program for 50 to 100 Patients

	No. Patients					
Cost Item	50	60	70	80	90	100
Nicotine gum (variable cost)	10,000	12,000	14,000	16,000	18,000	20,000
Pharmacist salary	26,000	26,000	26,000	26,000	26,000	26,000
Renovation	1,000	1,000	1,000	1,000	1,000	1,000
Training	100	100	100	100	100	100
Promotion	500	500	500	500	500	500
Indirect costs	500	500	500	500	500	500
Total fixed costs	28,100	28,100	28,100	28,100	28,100	28,100
Total costs	38,100	40,100	42,100	44,100	46,100	48,100
Cost per patient	762	668	601	551	512	481
Required profit per patient	13	11	9	8	7	7
Required price per patient	775	679	611	560	520	488

- A pharmacist will be hired to operate the smoking cessation clinic. The clinic will operate for 10 hours per week, and the pharmacist will staff the clinic (and be paid) for 10 hours per week regardless of patient volume. The pharmacist's salary, including benefits, will be $50 per hour.
- The pharmacy will be renovated to provide a private counseling area for the clinic. The renovation will cost $5,000 and will be depreciated over 5 years. Thus, the annual renovation-related expense will be $1,000.
- The pharmacy will spend $500 per year to promote the smoking cessation service.
- Training the pharmacist to provide behavioral counseling will cost $500. This will be depreciated over 5 years, giving an annual training expense of $100.
- The cost of nicotine gum will average $200 per patient.
- The clinic's share of indirect costs (such as insurance, manager's salary, rent, and utilities) will be $500 per year.

Most of the costs of operating the smoking cessation service are fixed costs, that is, costs that do not change as sales volume changes. The cost of the nicotine gum is a variable cost. As the number of patients served increases, the cost of nicotine gum increases proportionately.

To calculate average cost, the manager must have an estimate of the number of patients to be served. Her best guess is that the service will treat between 50 and 100 patients over the coming year. It is common for a manager not to know the exact level of demand for a new service but to be able to confidently estimate the range in which demand will fall. In such a case, the best practice is to estimate total and average costs across the full range of demand. The estimation of costs for the smoking cessation clinic for a range of demand between 50 and 100 patients is shown in Table 12-2. The pharmacy must charge at least $762 per patient to break even on the service at a volume of 50 patients. Charging less than $762 will result in a loss. However, if the volume is 100 patients, the pharmacy can charge $481 per patient and break even. As is true for most services, the average cost of providing the service declines as patient volume increases. This is a direct result of having substantial fixed costs.

STRATEGY FOR PRICING PHARMACIST SERVICES

A pharmacy needs an overall strategy for setting proper prices. The strategy should ensure that prices are high enough, in aggregate, to cover costs and a reasonable profit. At the same time, the strategy must recognize

TABLE 12-3   Estimated Demand for Smoking Cessation Services

Price per Patient ($)	No. Patients Purchasing Service
800	60
700	70
600	80
500	100
450	120

that the pharmacy's prices are constrained by its objectives, consumers, and competitors. The manager should keep in mind that the goal is to estimate the service's value to consumers and price it accordingly.

Estimate Demand

The manager's first step is to estimate consumer demand for the service. This consists of determining how much of the service consumers will purchase over a range of possible prices. Methods of estimating demand are discussed by Nagle and Holden,[2] Simon,[3] and Carroll.[4] The manager must remember that the demand for the service is influenced by all elements of the marketing mix, not just the price. An estimate of the demand for the smoking cessation service at Old City Pharmacy is shown in Table 12-3.

Calculate Cost of Providing Service

Then, the manager should calculate the pharmacy's cost of providing the service. This is the sum of the service cost and the costs of any materials or products needed to provide the service. Calculating the cost of providing the service lets the manager know how much, on average, the pharmacy must charge for each unit of service to break even. Because costs depend on volume, the manager should calculate the cost of providing the service over a range of sales volume. (Table 12-2 shows the estimated per patient costs of providing smoking cessation services.)

Determine Net Income

Next, the manager must determine the average amount of net income the pharmacy must make on each unit of service to meet its overall profit objective. The profit objective is based on the pharmacy's desired return on assets, then adjusted for competition, demand, and the pharmacy's objectives.

Old City Pharmacy has $5,500 invested in store renovation and pharmacist training to provide smoking cessation services. A reasonable goal would be to obtain a 12% return on these assets. To do so, the pharmacy would have to realize an annual profit of $660 ($5,500 × 0.12) on the service. The average, or per patient, profit required would be $660 divided by the number of patients served. If 50 patients were served, profit per patient would be set at $13.20 ($660/50). As with cost, the average, or per unit, profit depends on the volume of service sold. Table 12-2 presents estimates of the per patient profit required to meet the pharmacy's profit objective over the range of expected demand.

The amount of profit that is reasonable depends on the pharmacy's objectives and strategy. If it is following a penetration strategy, it may want to forgo all profits initially to increase sales more rapidly. If it has a skimming strategy, it will seek a higher profit.

Set Initial Price

The sum of the cost of providing the service and the average profit yields the initial set of prices the manager will consider. At a volume of 50 patients, the average cost of providing smoking cessation services is $762 and the desired net income is $13. The initial price to be considered for the service is the sum, or $775. As with costs and profits, the initial price to be considered should be calculated over the range of potential sales. Table 12-2 shows this calculation for Old City Pharmacy.

Compare Prices

The manager has now calculated the price that must be charged to make a profit on the service over a range of sales. He has also estimated demand—the quantity of service that consumers will purchase at each price. At this point, the manager compares the prices required to make a profit at each level of patient volume (or sales) with the prices needed to generate those levels of volume (or sales). The manager would like to see that at each level of price, the number of patients necessary to provide that price is lower than the number who will purchase the service at that price. The information for Old City Pharmacy in Table 12-2 and Table 12-3 indicates that patient demand will be sufficient to generate a profit at the initially estimated prices.

If the number of patients on which the price is based is higher than the number of patients who will demand the service at that price, then there is a problem; the pharmacy cannot profitably offer the service at a price patients are willing to pay. The manager has two options. First, he could conclude that the service is unprofitable and decide not to offer it.

Second, he could reexamine the costs of providing the service to find ways to reduce costs to a level that would allow the pharmacy to profitably offer the service at a price consumers would be willing to pay. If Old City Pharmacy had had this problem, it might have considered using staff pharmacists to provide the service rather than hiring an additional pharmacist. This would have lowered its costs at lower levels of demand.

For a new service, the manager must also keep in mind that volume may initially be low because consumers are not familiar with the service. Over time, demand should grow as consumers become more familiar with the service. This will occur if the pharmacy promotes the service, provides it in a manner that is convenient for consumers, and provides it in such a way that patients can see its value. Because of the cost–price–volume relationship, managers need to account for this initial period of low sales when estimating costs and setting initial prices. Specifically, if costs are based on the initial low volume, then prices may be set too high. Fewer consumers will purchase the service at these high prices.

Managers would do better to calculate costs, and set prices, on the basis of estimates of what sales volume will be after the service has become more familiar to consumers. This will lead to calculation of lower costs and prices, which, in turn, will result in higher sales of the service. Although the pharmacy will incur short-term losses on the service, this strategy prevents the manager from overpricing and killing demand for a service that would be profitable once consumers were familiar with it.

Consider Competitors' Responses

The manager must now consider how competitors will react to the service's price. A very low price might result in competitors lowering their prices. A high price could result in competitors aggressively promoting their lower prices.

Implement the Price

At this point, the manager is ready to offer the service at the decided-upon price.

Monitor Patient and Competitor Response

A service's price is based on estimates of demand, costs, and competitors' responses. After the price is set, the manager should carefully measure and document the actual response of patients and competitors to the service. Lower than anticipated demand may require lowering the price, increasing promotion, or re-evaluating the way the service is provided. Higher demand may allow raising the price to maximize profits or to limit demand to what the pharmacy can physically accommodate. The important point is that managers need to carefully monitor sales and competitors' responses to ensure that problems are quickly identified and addressed.

Re-evaluate

The manager must periodically evaluate prices to ensure that the service is generating its desired sales and profit. The price should be re-examined at least as often as the pharmacy's costs and competition change.

PRESENTING SERVICE PRICES TO CONSUMERS

Once an overall pricing strategy has been selected, several methods are available for presenting prices to buyers of pharmacist services.

Time and Expenses

Many pharmacists bill for their services on the basis of time and expenses. The pharmacist's charge is based directly on the time it takes to provide the service plus the costs of any out-of-pocket expenses incurred. Typically, the number of hours required to provide the service is multiplied by some constant that is large enough to cover the pharmacy's salary costs and overhead and yield a reasonable profit. A consultant pharmacist might charge a long-term care facility for doing drug regimen reviews for its patients according to the number of hours he spent conducting the reviews plus the number of miles he had to drive to reach the facility. The charge might be presented, for example, as $50 per hour spent reviewing charts plus 35 cents per mile driven. In this situation, the pricing problem is to determine the size of the constant that provides value for the customer and profit for the pharmacy.

Resource-Based Relative Value Scale

A variation of the time and expenses method is the resource-based relative value scale (RBRVS). In general, the RBRVS method bases the charges for a service on both the time spent providing the service and the intensity of effort required. The Peters Institute of Pharmaceutical Care at the University of Minnesota has proposed a RBRVS for pharmacist services.[8] The Peters Institute RBRVS allows the pharmacist to charge a purchaser of services according to the level of drug-related needs of the patient. The level of payment depends on six variables: the pharmacist's work-up, the pharmacist's assessment, the level of care planning and evaluation, the nature (risk) of the presenting drug therapy problems, counseling and coordination of care, and the face-to-face time involved in the encounter. These variables reflect the level of the patient's drug-related needs and, consequently, the time and intensity of pharmacist services required by the patient.

Fixed Fee

Another method of presenting or billing for services is to charge a fixed fee. A consultant pharmacist using this method might charge the long-term care facility a set monthly fee, say $500, for conducting drug regimen reviews on all patients at the facility. In our example, Old City Pharmacy estimated a fixed fee that it would charge each patient for providing a course of smoking cessation therapy.

Contingency Pricing

In some situations, pharmacists might bill for services on a contingency basis. In this method, the pharmacist's fee is based on a percentage of the savings that the pharmacist generates for the payer. PAID Prescriptions (a company that administers third-party prescription programs) at one time reimbursed pharmacies in its Coordinated Care Network 20% of the savings they generated through generic substitution. The contingency method has also been suggested as a way of charging third-party payers for pharmacist services. Essentially, the pharmacist's fees would be based on how much the service saved the third-party payer in total medical payments. This assumes that the service's contribution to better patient health will lead to lower costs for physician and hospital care. This method directly relates the value to the payer to the price of the service. On the other hand, it overlooks the value that patients receive from these services in ways that do not decrease medical costs. Patient-oriented services may improve patients' health, functioning, and satisfaction without decreasing medical costs.

Bundling

Price bundling involves selling a group, or bundle, of products and services as a package at one price. Bundling is a common practice. Computers and software are frequently sold together as a bundle. Dell computers, for example, come equipped with Microsoft Office software. Appliance dealers may bundle sale, delivery, and installation of new appliances for one price. Health maintenance organizations bundle all medical services together and sell them to consumers for a fixed monthly premium.

Pharmacies could bundle patient care services with related prescription products. In our example, Old City Pharmacy bundled smoking cessation counseling with nicotine gum.

Pharmacies have begun to administer immunizations to patients. Pharmacies typically provide the drug product and administer it to the patient at one price. This is another example of bundling. Pharmacists have offered this service to employer groups. In these situations, the pharmacist goes to the employer's workplace, discusses the importance of immunizations with groups of employees, then provides immunization to those employees who want it. Pharmacists could charge the employer a single, bundled price for the visit, education, provision of the product, and administration to employees.

To be successful, the bundle must offer the consumer more value than would purchasing the individual items in the bundle separately. Frequently, the bundle is offered at a lower price than that at which the consumer could purchase the items individually. In some instances, the bundle offers the consumer greater convenience. Selling computers and software together may not result in a lower price to the consumer, but it simplifies shopping, setup, and installation. In other instances, the business can produce the bundle of products less expensively than it can produce the individual components of the bundle.

Bundling is also useful when it improves the performance of products or services. In 1990, Sandoz (now a part of Novartis) offered its schizophrenia drug clozapine only as part of a bundled package that included mandatory weekly blood testing.[9] The bundle could be purchased only through two companies that provided both the drug and the blood tests. The two companies were selected on the basis that they would not dispense weekly refills of the drug until they received the patient's blood test results, and because they had their own facilities for doing blood tests. Sandoz set up this system because clozapine use had been linked to agranulocytosis, a rapid and sometimes fatal lowering of white blood cell counts. To ensure early detection of this condition in clozapine patients, Sandoz wanted a system that guaranteed that blood tests would be done weekly. Community pharmacists might consider bundling asthma, diabetes, and smoking cessation treatments with the counseling, monitoring, and educational services required to ensure that these products work as intended.

Capitation

Pharmacies have traditionally been paid by individual consumers and by third-party payers on a fee-for-service basis. With fee-for-service reimbursement, the pharmacy receives a separate payment for every unit of product or service provided. It is paid a fee for each prescription dispensed; the more prescriptions it dispenses, the more it is paid.

Some third-party payers have tried replacing fee-for-service reimbursement with capitation. Under the capitation method, patients enroll with a specific pharmacy (or group of pharmacies) and agree to get all of their pharmacist services and pharmacy products from that pharmacy (or group). The pharmacy is paid a predetermined monthly fee for each patient enrolled. The fee is the same regardless of how many, or how few, prescriptions and services the patient gets during each month. For example, long-term care pharmacies could be reimbursed on a capitated basis. If the capitation rate were $100, then the long-term care pharmacy would receive $100 per month for each patient in the facility. It would receive the same rate for each patient whether the patient received no prescriptions during the month or 12 prescriptions.

SUMMARY

Price is an important component of the marketing mix. In a sense, price reflects the value of all elements of the marketing mix. The manager's goal is to determine a price that will be profitable for the pharmacy and will provide good value to consumers.

References

1. Dolan RJ. How do you know when the price is right? *Harv Bus Rev.* 1995;73: 174–83.
2. Nagle TT, Holden RK. *The Strategy and Tactics of Pricing: A Guide to Profitable Decision Making.* 3rd ed. Upper Saddle River, NJ: Prentice Hall; 2002.
3. Simon H. Pricing opportunities—and how to exploit them. *Sloan Manage Rev.* 1992;33:55–65.
4. Carroll NV. Budgeting. In: *Financial Management for Pharmacists: A Decision-Making Approach.* Baltimore: Lippincott Williams & Wilkins; 2007;77–98.
5. Zeithaml VA, Bitner MJ. Pricing of services. In: *Services Marketing.* New York: McGraw-Hill; 1996:482–515.
6. Chain Pharmacy Industry Profile, 2006. Alexandria, Va: NACDS Foundation; 2006.
7. Carroll NV. Pricing pharmaceutical products and services. In: *Financial Management for Pharmacists: A Decision Making Approach.* Baltimore: Lippincott Williams & Wilkins; 2007:123–54.
8. Cipolle RJ, Strand LM, Morley PC. A reimbursement system for pharmaceutical care. In: *Pharmaceutical Care Practice.* New York: McGraw Hill; 1998:267–96.
9. Salzman C. Mandatory monitoring for side effects: the "bundling" of clozapine. *N Engl J Med.* 1990;323:827–30.

Additional Readings

Christensen DB, Fassett WE. Understanding capitation and pharmaceutical care. *J Am Pharm Assoc.* 1996;NS36:374-80.

Kotler P, Bloom PN. Setting fees. In: *Marketing Professional Services.* Englewood Cliffs, NJ: Prentice Hall; 1984.

Tellis GJ. Beyond the many faces of price: an integration of pricing strategies. *J Mark.* 1986;50:146-60.

Exercises and Questions

1. Why should pricing be based on value to the consumer rather than cost to the pharmacy?
2. Consider cosmetic surgery and heart surgery to repair blocked arteries. For which would demand be more elastic? Why?
3. Why might pharmacies offering warfarin monitoring services not want to offer low prices for the service?
4. List and discuss five services that pharmacies could offer to decrease consumers' time, search, and psychic costs.
5. Wal-Mart recently began to offer a wide variety of generic prescription products for $4 for a monthly supply. What was Wal-Mart's objective in doing this? How does Wal-Mart expect to profit from this practice?
6. In what situation could a pharmacy begin by offering prices that were below its costs and end up being profitable without raising its prices? (Hint: Consider the interdependency of cost, volume, and price.)
7. Joe's Professional Pharmacy would like to begin to offer a diabetes counseling and monitoring service. How could it structure the service so that the salaries associated with the service were direct costs? How could it structure the service so that salaries were indirect costs?

CHAPTER 13

CHANNELS OF DISTRIBUTION

By Norman V. Carroll, PhD

Professor of Pharmacy Administration
Virginia Commonwealth University School of Pharmacy

Objectives

After studying this chapter, the reader should be able to

❏ Define and give examples of a channel of distribution for pharmacy products and services.
❏ Define and give examples of members of channels of distribution for pharmacy products and services.
❏ Define the term intermediary, give examples of intermediaries, and list and describe the functions intermediaries fulfill in channels of distribution.
❏ Discuss the effects of customer, product, and manufacturer characteristics on channel structure and explain why different types of pharmacy products and services require different channel structures.
❏ Define and give examples of channel conflict and cooperation.
❏ List and explain the types of vertical marketing systems and discuss the need for them.
❏ Explain the functions and services offered by pharmacy benefit managers and the effects these organizations have had on community pharmacy.
❏ Explain how the growth of managed care has led to increasing cooperation and consolidation among pharmacy retailers and increasing conflict between retailers and other channel members.

Channels of distribution are the paths through which goods, and information and payment for those goods, travel on their way from manufacturer to ultimate consumer. A channel of distribution consists of the producer of the good, the ultimate user, and any middlemen through which the goods pass. A typical channel of distribution for a pharmacy product consists of the manufacturer (e.g., Merck or Pfizer), a pharmaceutical wholesaler (e.g., McKesson or Cardinal), a community pharmacy, and the patient who ultimately receives the product.

> *A channel of distribution consists of the producer of the good, the ultimate user, and any middlemen through which the goods pass.*

Channels of distribution for services tend to be much shorter. Services are usually produced and consumed simultaneously, so they cannot be stocked or shipped to other locations. The typical channel for provision of a service is producer to consumer. For example, the pharmacist produces smoking cessation services at the same time the patient consumes those services. Although the channel for providing services is usually short, the channel for paying for the service or for providing information about the service can be lengthy.

CHANNEL MEMBERS

A *manufacturer* is a business that produces a finished product from raw materials. Examples of pharmaceutical manufacturers are Merck, Pfizer, and Barr Laboratories. The pharmaceutical industry has two basic types of manufacturers. Research-oriented manufacturers not only manufacture drug products, they also conduct research to discover and develop new drugs. The Pharmaceutical Research and Manufacturers of America (PhRMA), which is the trade group representing the research-oriented manufacturers, has 32 members with sales in the United States of $164 billion in 2005.[1] A growing sector of the research-oriented pharmaceutical industry is biotechnology. In 2005 there were 1,415 biotechnology companies in the United States, according to the Biotechnology Industry Organization (BIO).[2] BIO member companies reported sales of $50.7 billion in 2005. (Some companies are members of both PhRMA and BIO.) The second type of manufacturer is the generic drug company. Generic companies manufacture products that are no longer protected by patents. They spend relatively little on research and development. Generic drug companies outnumber research-oriented companies, but they are much smaller organizations. U.S. retail sales of generic drugs amounted to $22.3 billion in 2005.[3]

A *wholesaler* is a business that purchases finished goods for resale to other businesses. Wholesalers do not sell to ultimate consumers. Pharmaceutical wholesalers, such as AmerisourceBergen and McKesson, purchase prescription and nonprescription products from manufacturers and sell them to retailers. The Healthcare Distribution Management Association (HDMA), the trade group representing pharmaceutical wholesalers, had 46 full-service member companies that operated 155 distribution centers in the United States in 2005.[4] About 59% of all prescription products sold in the United States are distributed through wholesalers,[5] and 68% of prescription products sold at chain drugstores are distributed through chain pharmacy warehouses. The pharmaceutical wholesaling industry is dominated by three large wholesalers: McKesson, AmerisourceBergen, and Cardinal Health.

Retailers are businesses that purchase finished goods for resale to, or use by, ultimate consumers. In the vocabulary of distribution channels, pharmaceutical retailers include hospital pharmacies, in-house health maintenance organization (HMO) pharmacies, long-term care pharmacies, clinics, and mail order pharmacies, as well as chain and independent community pharmacies. All of these are classified as retailers because they furnish products directly to the ultimate consumer. Table 13-1[6] shows the percentages of all prescription products sold through various types of pharmacy retailers.

TABLE 13-1 Pharmaceutical Retailers by Share of Total Prescription Drug Sales, United States

Retailer Type	% Market Share
Pharmacies	
Chain stores	28.1
Independents	13.7
Mail order	14.6
Mass merchandisers	6.9
Supermarkets	8.5
Total community pharmacy	71.8
Providers	
Hospitals	11.8
Clinics	9.8
Long-term care	4.8
Miscellaneous[a]	1.9
Total providers	28.3

[a] Includes home health care, health maintenance organizations, and others.

Source: Reference 6.

FIGURE 13-1 Interactions between manufacturers and consumers in a channel with no retailers.

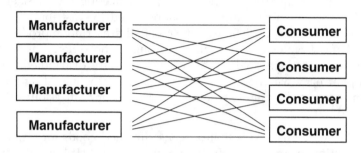

INTERMEDIARIES IN CHANNELS OF DISTRIBUTION

Wholesalers and retailers are referred to as *intermediaries*. In most channel structures, manufacturers use intermediaries to distribute their products. Intermediaries are used when they increase the efficiency of channels and when they can provide services that are difficult or not economical for manufacturers to provide.

Intermediaries improve the efficiency of distribution channels by decreasing the number of required interactions between members of the channel. A simple example shows how this works. Assume that a distribution channel consists of four manufacturers and four consumers. If each consumer makes a purchase of each manufacturer's product every week, then 16 interactions are required between consumers and manufacturers each week (Figure 13-1). Each consumer must deal with each of the four manufacturers each week. If one retailer is introduced into the channel, the number of total weekly contacts drops from 16 to 8; the number of contacts for each consumer drops to 1 (Figure 13-2). The pharmaceutical industry consists of hundreds of manufacturers and millions of ultimate consumers. Pharmaceutical wholesalers and retailers dramatically improve the efficiency of drug distribution. HDMA estimates that pharmaceutical wholesalers cut the annual number of transactions between manufacturers and pharmacies from 4.5 billion (if there were no wholesalers) to 34.8 million.[7]

Intermediaries are also used when manufacturers lack the resources to perform all the functions necessary to adequately provide their products to consumers. Advantages provided by intermediaries include the following:

- *Increased convenience.* Pharmaceutical wholesalers and retailers provide pharmacy products at places and times that are convenient for

FIGURE 13-2 Interactions between manufacturers and consumers in a channel with a retailer.

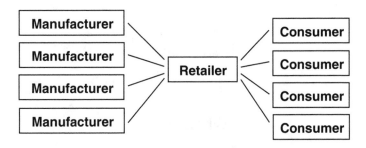

consumers. For a consumer in North Dakota who needs a product made by GlaxoSmithKline, it is much more convenient to purchase the product at a local pharmacy than to purchase it from the manufacturing plant in North Carolina.

- *Variety.* Intermediaries provide a broad assortment of products; consumers can conveniently purchase products made by many manufacturers from one retailer or wholesaler. It is more convenient for pharmacies to deal with one wholesaler than with the hundreds of manufacturers whose products they stock. The typical pharmaceutical wholesaler deals with an average of 670 manufacturers.[4]
- *Services.* One important service that intermediaries provide is breaking large packages into smaller sizes that are more appropriate for consumers' needs. Wholesalers buy products by the case and sell them to pharmacies by the bottle. Pharmacies buy bottles of hundreds or thousands and dispense the products to patients in bottles of fives, thirties, or sixties. Many intermediaries also provide credit and delivery services to customers. Pharmacies provide their patients with information about the proper use of pharmacy products; much of this information—such as proper use of inhalers and glucometers—is better provided by pharmacists face-to-face than by manufacturers through printed information. In addition, a pharmacist can tailor the information provided to individual patients, while manufacturers must provide a standardized set of instructions for all consumers.

FACTORS INFLUENCING CHANNEL STRUCTURE

Channel structure develops to fit the needs and characteristics of the customer, product, and manufacturer. The typical channel of distribution for pharmacy products is shown in Figure 13-3. This is a long channel because it includes two intermediaries. Not all channels share this structure. In fact, not all channels for pharmacy products share this structure. A number of factors determine the channel structure.

FIGURE 13-3 Typical channel of distribution for a pharmaceutical product. Solid arrows represent goods; dashed arrows represent payment.

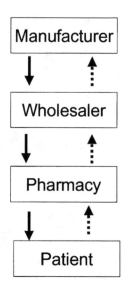

Customer Characteristics

Pharmaceutical manufacturers use both wholesalers and retailers because they have a large number of customers—thousands of pharmacies and hundreds of millions of consumers, because their customers are dispersed across the world, and because their customers make relatively small and frequent purchases. It would be prohibitively expensive for a manufacturer to establish its own distribution channel to serve this many customers in this many different locations.

Manufacturers of other types of products have developed different channels. For example, the channels of distribution for nuclear submarines are short; they consist of only manufacturer and consumer. One reason for this is their customer characteristics: There are very few customers (governments of a few nations), they are in a few readily identifiable areas (the capitals of those nations), and they make large and infrequent purchases. Consequently, it is efficient and more effective for the manufacturer to deal directly with the ultimate consumer.

Product Characteristics

Most pharmacy products share a number of characteristics that allow them to have long distribution channels. First, most are sufficiently nonperishable that they can be shipped and stored for extended periods of time. In comparison, products such as milk and eggs need shorter channels because they do not last long enough to allow them to be shipped to and held by intermediaries. Pharmacy products are not bulky, so it is economical to ship and store them. Shipping and storage are greater problems for products like iron ore and coal. Because pharmacy products are standardized, they can be sold and resold without detailed inspection. In contrast, nonstandardized products, such as livestock and uncut diamonds, must be inspected and graded each time they are sold. Finally, most pharmacy products have low unit value, so wholesalers and retailers can afford to hold inventories of these products. Holding inventories of very expensive products, such as airplanes, is much less feasible.

Some pharmacy products require short channels. Nuclear pharmacy products have extremely short half-lives, so it is not feasible to store them. Compounded products typically have short channels because they are made for a specific patient. In addition, pharmacist services have short channels because it is not possible to store or ship them.

Manufacturer Characteristics

Pharmaceutical manufacturers offer limited product lines. No manufacturer has a sufficiently broad line of pharmacy products that it can serve all consumers. As a result, manufacturers need intermediaries that will buy from many manufacturers and offer consumers a proper assortment of products. Pharmaceutical manufacturers also serve national and international markets; serving these markets requires many outlets.

CHANNEL RELATIONSHIPS

A channel of distribution consists of a number of organizations, each with its own goals and objectives. In pursuing their goals, organizations frequently find themselves in conflict with other organizations in the channel. At other times, they may cooperate with the other organizations to reach mutual goals.

Conflict in the Channel

When conflict between channel members occurs, it impairs the efficiency and effectiveness of the channel. There are many examples of conflict in pharmaceutical channels.

As one example, in 1994 a large number of independent and chain community pharmacies sued the major research-oriented pharmaceutical manufacturers over preferential pricing[8,9]—the practice of charging different prices to different types of pharmacies for the same products in the same quantities. The research-oriented pharmaceutical companies charge lower prices to managed care organizations (MCOs) and mail order pharmacies and substantially higher prices to community pharmacies. They argue that it is in their best interests to do so because MCOs and mail order pharmacies have the ability to "move market share." That is, they argue that these entities use formularies and therapeutic interchange programs to increase sales of one manufacturer's products at the expense of competitors' products. If they did not offer lower prices to MCOs and mail order pharmacies, these organizations would not use their products. The drug companies also argue that they do not discount prices to community pharmacies because those pharmacies do not have the ability to move market share. Community pharmacies argue that the research-oriented manufacturers have never given them the opportunity to gain discounts for moving market share and that, in fact, the manufacturers have illegally conspired as a group to keep them from getting discounts. The conflict has resulted in ill will, lack of trust, and substantial legal expense for both manufacturers and retailers, and has still not been resolved.

Another pharmacy-related example is dispensing generic drugs for prescriptions written for chemically identical brand-name products. MCOs support and encourage the use of generic products because generics are substantially cheaper than brand-name drugs. MCOs have numerous programs to increase the use of generic drugs.[10–13] The research-oriented companies that produce brand-name drugs are opposed to such use of generics because it decreases their sales and profits. Since the mid-1950s, brand-name manufacturers have resisted the use of generic drugs through lobbying, influencing legislation, and legal actions.[14–17]

There has also been conflict over the limited distribution of drug products such as clozapine[18] and alendronate,[19] the use of restricted formularies in state Medicaid programs and MCOs,[20,21] and the proper role of industry detailers in MCOs and hospitals.[22] These conflicts have impaired the smooth functioning of the distribution channel by consuming time and effort that could have been better spent serving patients.

Cooperation in the Channel

Cooperation by channel members usually increases the efficiency and effectiveness of the channel so that all channel members benefit. *Buying groups* (or *group purchasing organizations [GPOs]*) are one example of channel cooperation in pharmacy. A buying group pools the purchasing power of a large number of individual pharmacies in order to extract better prices from suppliers. The members of a buying group must agree to make all (or a high percentage) of their purchases of contracted items from the supplier selected by the group. Because of the volume of sales involved, the supplier is much more likely to provide lower prices to the buying group than to individual pharmacies.

Buying groups have become quite prevalent. The Health Industry Group Purchasing Association, the trade association for GPOs, estimates that 96% to 98% of hospitals use a GPO.[23] Most hospital pharmacies are members of buying groups, and buying groups for other types of pharmacies are also common. The Federation of Pharmacy Networks is composed of 22 buying groups that represent 13,000 independent pharmacies.[24] According to the *Managed Care Digest,* 72% of HMOs with in-house pharmacies use buying groups.[25] Examples of pharmacy-related buying groups include EPIC and PACE Alliance for independent pharmacies and Novation and Premier for hospitals.

A *prime vendor* arrangement is a similar example of cooperation. In a prime vendor system a group of pharmacies, such as a buying group, agrees to make the majority of its purchases through a single wholesaler. This wholesaler is designated as the group's prime vendor. In return for the assured business, the wholesaler discounts its normal price to the participating pharmacies.

Buying groups are examples of cooperation at the same level of distribution; they are examples of cooperation among retailers. There can also be cooperation between different levels of distribution; one example is the *charge-back system* that allows manufacturers to distribute products at preferential prices through wholesalers.

As mentioned previously, pharmaceutical manufacturers charge different prices to different types of pharmacies. Most pharmaceutical manufacturers find it more efficient to distribute their products through wholesalers. The problem that manufacturers face is how to charge different prices to different types of pharmacies and, at the same time, sell these products through a wholesaler.

The problem is solved by the charge-back system. In this system, manufacturers sell all of their products to wholesalers at a set price, for example, average wholesale price (AWP) less 20%. The wholesaler then sells to pharmacies at prices negotiated between the pharmacies and the manufacturers. The wholesaler might charge community pharmacies AWP minus 15%, long-term care pharmacies AWP minus 25%, and HMO pharmacies AWP minus 35%. In this example, the wholesaler would make a gross profit of 5% of AWP on products sold to community pharmacies. However, it would lose 5% on sales to long-term care pharmacies and 15% on sales to HMO pharmacies. To cover the losses, the wholesaler would inform the manufacturer about its quantity of sales to each type of pharmacy and charge the manufacturer an amount sufficient to provide a 5% profit on sales to long-term care and HMO pharmacies.

The operation of this system requires close cooperation between wholesaler and manufacturer. The wholesaler must agree to abide by the manufacturer's price agreements with retailers and provide detailed information to the manufacturer about its sales to each type of pharmacy. The manufacturer must make its prices to retailers known to the wholesalers and establish a system for efficiently managing the charge-back information from wholesalers and for paying them in a reasonable amount of time. The two parties are willing to participate in this arrangement because it allows each party to meet its individual goals.

Vertical Marketing Systems

Because of the efficiencies of cooperation, various forms of *vertical marketing systems* have arisen. Vertical marketing systems provide more efficient and effective channels, because one channel member manages the channel to increase cooperation and decrease conflict. This channel member is known as the *channel captain*. There are three basic types of vertical marketing systems.

In *administered systems,* there is no formal agreement among members of the channel. Instead, one member of the channel, because of its greater power, administers the channel. This member is the channel captain. Because of their size and financial strength, the large, research-oriented pharmaceutical manufacturers have traditionally administered channels of distribution for patented pharmacy products. These companies exercise channel leadership by making, or strongly influencing, decisions about pricing, promotion, and distribution of patented pharmacy products.

Manufacturers are not the channel captains in all administered systems. In mass merchandising, the retailer is more likely to be the channel captain. Wal-Mart, for example, controls the channels of distribution for most products sold in its stores. This is because Wal-Mart is larger and financially stronger than most of its suppliers.

In *corporate systems,* a single corporation owns and operates all levels of distribution—manufacturer, wholesaler, and retailer—within the system. Sherwin Williams Paint is a corporate vertical marketing system. Sherwin Williams makes its own paints, distributes them through its own warehouses, and sells to consumers through its own retail stores.

For 10 years, Merck owned a corporate system for pharmacy products. Merck develops and manufactures pharmacy products in its research laboratories and production facilities. From 1993 to 2003, it owned Medco, a company that owned both a mail order pharmacy and PAID Prescriptions (a pharmacy benefit manager). Merck products were distributed through Medco's mail order pharmacy and through pharmacies that had contracts with PAID Prescriptions. (Medco is now an independent company.) Cardinal Health, a major pharmaceutical wholesaler, has a partial corporate system. Cardinal owns the Medicine Shoppe franchise of community pharmacies. Thus, Cardinal can distribute its products through its own community pharmacies. (Cardinal also sells products, and realizes most of its sales volume, through outlets it does not own.)

Integrated health care systems are also corporate systems. In these systems, one member of the channel, usually the hospital, owns physician practices, hospitals, and pharmacies. Thus, one corporation provides all elements of medical care.

The third type of vertical marketing system is a *contractual system*. In these, the channel captain licenses or franchises other channel members to use its products, services, signs, and logos. One example of a contractual system in pharmacy is a *wholesaler-sponsored voluntary chain*. The major pharmaceutical wholesalers have organized voluntary chains of independent pharmacies. Pharmacies in these chains agree to use a common logo and signage, to participate in wholesaler-sponsored purchasing programs for generic drugs and private-label nonprescription merchandise, and to participate in group advertising and promotional programs. Some of the voluntary chains also negotiate and administer third-party contracts as a group under the sponsorship of the chain. For example, AmerisourceBergen sponsors the Good Neighbor Pharmacies voluntary chain. Pharmacies that are part of the chain display the Good Neighbor logo on signs inside and outside the pharmacy, purchase generic and private-label nonprescription goods through AmerisourceBergen, and promote themselves through wholesaler-coordinated advertising programs that identify them as Good Neighbor Pharmacies. Advertising as a group makes it economically feasible for the pharmacies to advertise in media, such as regional newspapers, radio, and television, that would be too expensive for individual pharmacies to use.

The voluntary chain structure provides independent pharmacies with economies of scale in purchasing, advertising, and managed care contracting similar to those enjoyed by large chain pharmacies. In addition, the sponsoring wholesalers may provide such services as Web-site development, merchandising and management assistance, and disease management programs. Wholesalers sponsor these chains because it promotes the financial viability of their independent pharmacy customers and ties these customers more closely to the wholesaler. Table 13-2[26-31] lists the major wholesaler-sponsored chains and their membership.

TABLE 13-2   Major Wholesaler-Sponsored Chains

Name of Chain	Sponsor	No. Member Pharmacies
Performance Plus Network	AmerisourceBergen	3,500
Leader Drug Stores	Cardinal Health	3,300
AccessHealth	McKesson	3,000
Health Mart	McKesson	3,000
Good Neighbor Pharmacy	AmerisourceBergen	2,500
Family Pharmacy	AmerisourceBergen	2,300

Sources: References 26–31.

CHANGES IN CHANNELS OF DISTRIBUTION FOR PHARMACY PRODUCTS AND SERVICES

The health care system has experienced significant change over the past two decades. The major driver of change has been the dramatic increase in health care spending. Total spending on health care in the United States grew from $75 billion in 1970 to $1.9 trillion in 2004.[32] Spending on pharmacy products at the retail level grew even faster, from $5.5 billion in 1970 to $189 billion in 2004.[32] As spending on health care has grown, the organizations that pay for health care—state and federal government and employers—have looked to managed care to bring health care spending under control. Managed care, according to Stefano and Navarro,[33] attempts to "control the cost, distribution, and utilization of health care products and services while providing high-quality health care to customers." One of the major means by which MCOs have attempted to control costs has been through negotiating discounts with drug makers and pharmacies.

As Figure 13-4 shows, the amount that pharmacies receive for dispensing third-party prescriptions has dropped over the past several years.[34] In 1996 the typical community pharmacy would have been reimbursed $90.37 for a prescription with a $100 AWP; in 2000 the pharmacy would have received $87.15. The situation is compounded by the growing proportion of prescriptions that are paid for by MCOs. As shown in Figure 13-5, 87% of retail prescriptions were reimbursed by third-party payers in 2005. (Almost all third-party payers are MCOs.) The resulting pressures on profits have led to a number of significant changes in the channels of distribution. The following sections discuss the major changes that have affected community pharmacy (Figure 13-6).

Pharmacy Benefit Managers

One of the most significant changes in channels of distribution has been the development and growth of pharmacy benefit managers (PBMs).

FIGURE 13-4 Changes in pharmacy reimbursement from employer-sponsored health plans. Dark bars are AWP discount, the percentage subtracted from average wholesale price to obtain the pharmacy reimbursement for drug product cost. Light bars are the dollar amounts of dispensing fees. (Compiled from reference 34.)

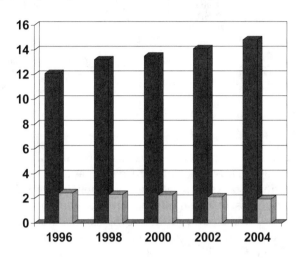

FIGURE 13-5 Percentages of retail prescriptions reimbursed by third-party payers. (Compiled from reference 6 and *American Druggist* annual prescription trends surveys, 1970–1995.)

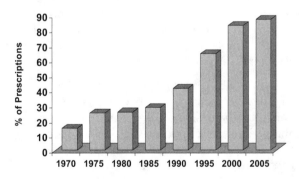

PBMs are organizations that contract with MCOs, insurance companies, and self-insured employers to manage their prescription drug benefit programs.

PBMs arose to meet the need to handle prescription claims and payments more efficiently. Since the mid-1980s, there has been tremendous

FIGURE 13-6 Changes in channels of distribution for prescription drugs at the retail level. PBMs = pharmacy benefit managers.

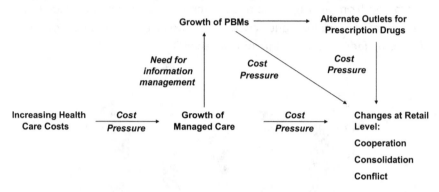

growth in the number of prescriptions that are reimbursed by third-party payers (Figure 13-5). The growth of third-party payment led to an increase in the administrative tasks associated with dispensing and obtaining payment for prescriptions. In a cash transaction, the pharmacist takes the prescription, checks it for accuracy and appropriateness, dispenses it to the patient, and collects payment from the patient. A third-party transaction is more complicated. In addition to the basic dispensing tasks, the pharmacist must ensure that the patient is covered by the third-party plan, ensure that the particular product prescribed and the supply prescribed are covered by the third party, and submit a claim for payment to the third party. Claims submission and payment became a significant problem, because each pharmacy submitted claims to hundreds of third-party plans and each self-insured employer, insurance company, or MCO remitted payments to thousands of pharmacies. PBMs developed to serve as intermediaries in claims processing. In essence, PBMs serve as wholesalers for prescription claims and payments (Figure 13-7).

Before we look at PBMs in more detail, some discussion of terminology is needed. The PBMs' customers are called *plan sponsors*. These are the MCOs, insurance companies, and self-insured employer groups that hire PBMs to manage their prescription drug plans. The consumers who are covered by plan sponsors' prescription drug plans are called *beneficiaries*, *members*, or *covered lives*. The specific details of coverage are called the *plan*.

PBMs serve as intermediaries between pharmacies and plan sponsors (Figure 13-7). A PBM receives claims from pharmacies, aggregates them by plan sponsor, and submits one aggregate claim to each plan sponsor. Each sponsor reimburses the PBM for the aggregate claim. The PBM collects payments from all its plan sponsors, aggregates payments by pharmacy, and reimburses individual pharmacies.

FIGURE 13-7 Function of pharmacy benefit manager (PBM) as whole-saler for prescription claims and payments. Solid arrows represent claims; dashed arrows represent payment.

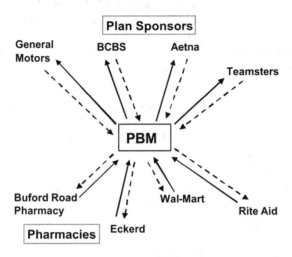

As with wholesalers in the product channel, PBMs add efficiency by cutting down the number of required interactions. Instead of receiving millions of claims from thousands of pharmacies every 2 weeks, a plan sponsor receives one bill and writes one check to its PBM. Rather than having to submit claims and receive payments from hundreds of plan sponsors every 2 weeks, a pharmacy submits claims and receives checks from a few PBMs.

An important part of a PBM's duties is the development of a *network* of retail pharmacies. A network consists of pharmacies that agree to dispense prescriptions to the plan sponsor's members. To become part of a network, pharmacies must agree to discount the prices they charge the plan sponsor. The price is typically established by the PBM as the AWP of the product less a percentage discount plus a dispensing fee. A typical reimbursement might be AWP minus 14% plus $2.

PBMs have also added efficiency to distribution channels by developing *on-line claims adjudication systems*. Before the implementation of these systems, pharmacies could never be sure if an individual was a member of a given third-party prescription plan, if the prescription product was covered by the plan, if there were any limitations on the supply dispensed, or what the proper co-payment should be. As a result, pharmacy claims were frequently denied or adjusted downward because the patient or drug was not covered, because an inappropriate quantity was dispensed, or because the wrong co-payment was collected. This led to significant conflict between pharmacies and PBMs. With on-line adjudication, the claim is electronically submitted to the PBM as the pharmacy is processing the prescription. The PBM immediately reviews the claim for appropriateness and sends an electronic message back to the pharmacy indicating whether the claim is accepted and what the co-payment should be. Because the system operates electronically, rapidly, and in real time, the pharmacist gets approval for the claim before the prescription is dispensed to the patient. This has substantially reduced the number of denied claims that pharmacies receive.

Over time, PBMs developed additional services to add value for plan sponsors. In response to the need for cost containment, most PBMs now offer to design and manage the prescription benefit for plan sponsors. PBMs offer programs and interventions to maximize the effectiveness and minimize the cost of drug therapy, such as drug-use review; utilization review and management (providing plan sponsors with reports showing utilization and expenditures by drug, class, pharmacy, and prescriber); physician education and counterdetailing; mail order programs; drug exclusions, quantity limits, and co-payments; formulary programs; and manufacturer rebate programs.

Today, PBMs are an integral part of the distribution channel for pharmacy products and services. Table 13-3 lists the major PBMs. As these numbers show, a majority of retail prescriptions in the United States are managed by PBMs, and about one-third are managed by one of the three largest PBMs.

TABLE 13-3 Largest Pharmacy Benefit Management (PBM) Companies

Company	2005 Prescription Volume (no. prescriptions)
Express Scripts	300,873,625
Caremark Prescription Services	387,514,842
Medco Health Solutions	397,223,877
Total for three largest PBMs	1,085,612,344
Total for all PBMs	1,766,835,776
Total retail volume	3,174,525,316

Source: Reference 6.

FIGURE 13-8 Growth of mail order pharmacies.
(Compiled from reference 6.)

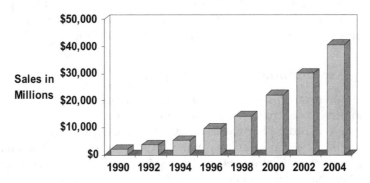

Alternative Retail Outlets for Prescription Drugs

The growth of managed care has encouraged the growth of a number of new types of retail outlets for prescription drugs. The largest growth has occurred among mail order pharmacies. As shown in Figure 13-8, the volume of prescription sales by mail order pharmacies has increased dramatically over the past several years. This has occurred primarily as a result of demand from plan sponsors.

PBMs promote distribution through mail order pharmacies as less costly to plan sponsors than distribution through community pharmacies.[35-37] Mail order pharmacies offer economies through efficient dispensing operations and through their preferential pricing from the pharmaceutical industry. (There is some evidence that, in spite of these advantages, mail order pharmacies do not yield lower costs to plan sponsors.[38-40]) The major PBMs encourage plan sponsors to use mail order because they own mail order pharmacies and make higher profits on prescriptions dispensed through them. PBMs and plan sponsors frequently design their drug benefit plans so that patients are given economic incentives to use mail order. For example, in 2005 the Virginia state employees prescription plan charged patient co-payments of $60 for a 90-day supply of a preferred brand-name product at a community pharmacy but only $40 for a 90-day supply of the same product from a mail order pharmacy.

There has also been a substantial increase in physician dispensing. Sales of pharmacy products through physicians' offices and clinics rose from $1.1 billion in 1990 to $24.7 billion in 2005.[6,41] This may be a result of increases in the number of urgent care clinics as well as the shift of care from inpatient to outpatient settings. Many urgent care clinics, such as Patient First, have their physicians dispense drugs to patients at the time of diagnosis and treatment. The shift of care from inpatient to outpatient settings has resulted in more injectable drugs, such as cancer chemotherapy, being administered in physicians' offices and clinics.

Changes in Community Pharmacy

The downward pressure that managed care discounting has exerted on community pharmacy prices and profits and the increased competition from mail order pharmacies and physician dispensing have changed the structure of community pharmacy. The changes can be characterized as cooperation with other retail pharmacies, consolidation, and conflict with other channel members.

Cooperation

In order to survive, independent pharmacies have had to increase the extent to which they cooperate with each other. Buying groups and wholesaler-sponsored voluntary chains are examples. Both types of arrangement require that independent pharmacies cooperate to realize economies in purchasing, advertising, or contracting with MCOs. Independent pharmacies need these efficiencies to compete with larger chains and to be able to survive on the declining prices paid by MCOs.

Over time, many buying groups have added functions that require further cooperation among pharmacies. Among the most common are group advertising and managed care contracting. In the latter case, pharmacies give the buying group the right to enter into managed care contracts on their behalf. In some cases, the buying group may also act as a PBM for its member pharmacies and plan sponsors. That is, the buying group collects claims and distributes payments to pharmacies so that each plan sponsor deals with only one organization. Buying groups (or other organizations) that administer third-party contracts for groups of pharmacies have been called *professional services administrative organizations* (PSAOs). An example is EPIC Pharmacies, which has several hundred pharmacy members in the Middle Atlantic States.

As discussed later, community pharmacies have also become more likely to cooperate with each other in bringing their problems to legislatures and courts.

At another level, the major trade groups representing community pharmacy—the National Association of Chain Drug Stores (NACDS) and the National Community Pharmacists Association (NCPA)—have begun to cooperate more closely to meet common goals. In 1998, the groups jointly founded the National Institute for Standards in Pharmacist Credentialing (NISPC).[42] The purpose of NISPC is to develop standards for testing and recognizing pharmacists' abilities to manage specific diseases. Another major joint effort has been the formation of the SureScript System.[43] The goal of this project is to establish direct and secure electronic communications between pharmacists and physicians. This will allow physicians to transmit electronic prescriptions to pharmacies, and physicians and pharmacists to communicate electronically about refills, drug-use review problems, and other patient care issues. In addition, NACDS and NCPA have developed a technician training manual and founded the Institute for the Advancement of Pharmaceutical Care, an organization that supports educational and research programs designed to enhance community pharmacy practice.

Consolidation

Pharmacies have been relatively powerless in their negotiations with MCOs because no one pharmacy, or pharmacy chain, has a dominant position in its geographic market. Added to this, PBMs have not perceived significant service differences among pharmacies. Put another way, MCOs and PBMs have regarded pharmacies as commodities. They have seen no reason to prefer one pharmacy to another in terms of service, so they have accepted any pharmacy that accepted their price. The result has been declining prices and profits for pharmacies.

The larger chain pharmacies have responded by consolidating. They have purchased independents and smaller chains and merged with each other to increase their market share. The result is fewer, but much larger, chains. As shown in Table 13-4,[6,44] in 1990 the four largest chains operated 7,379 pharmacies. This figure accounted for 41% of all chain pharmacies and 13% of all community pharmacies. By 2005, the four largest chains operated 15,499 pharmacies. This accounted for 73% of traditional chain pharmacies and 28% of all community pharmacies. Table 13-4 also shows that five of the nine largest chains in 1990 had been acquired by other chains by 2005. The large chain pharmacies may now be approaching the size and market presence required to negotiate prices with PBMs.

Larger size also makes the chains more attractive to PBMs. It is much simpler administratively for a PBM to deal with one large regional or national chain than to deal with several smaller chains or independents. (The wholesaler-sponsored chains and PSAOs began to offer managed care contracting services so that independents could offer PBMs the same administrative simplicity as chains.)

TABLE 13-4   Consolidation among Chain Pharmacies

Chain	No. Pharmacies in 1990	No. Pharmacies in 2000[a]	No. Pharmacies in 2005[a]
Rite Aid	2,352	3,800	3,323
Revco	1,870	(CVS)	(CVS)
Eckerd	1,632	2,898	1,853 (Brooks-Eckerd)
Walgreens	1,525	3,165	4,953
Hook-SuperX	1,110	(CVS)	(CVS)
Thrifty	1,065	(Rite Aid)	(Rite Aid)
CVS	801	4,082	5,370
Osco	672	(Albertson's)	(Albertson's)
Thrift Drug	472	(Eckerd)	(Brooks-Eckerd)
Total	11,499	13,945	15,499

[a] Parentheses indicate the chain has been acquired; the name in parentheses is the acquiring chain (e.g., Revco was acquired by CVS).

Sources: References 6 and 44.

A third benefit of consolidation is expense reduction resulting from economies of scale. At the organizational level, increasing the number of pharmacies in a chain can result in economies in purchasing, distribution, advertising, and administration. Chains also realize economies at the individual pharmacy level. Closing competing pharmacies in a consolidated chain can result in higher per store volume and the economies that come from operating closer to full capacity.

Conflict with Other Channel Members

Community pharmacies have become more likely to take their grievances to the courts and legislatures. In 1994, several chains and independent pharmacy groups sued the major research-oriented manufacturers and wholesalers, charging that they illegally colluded to fix prices and that preferential pricing was illegal.[8,9] Many of these cases have been resolved by a class action settlement.[45] However, a number of independent groups have continued their cases because the class settlement did not end the practice of preferential pricing.

Before implementation of the Medicare Part D drug program, NACDS and NCPA brought suit against the federal government to stop it from endorsing and supporting a PBM-based drug discount card for senior citizens.[46] One of the pharmacy organizations' major concerns with the plan was that any savings realized would come from lower reimbursements to pharmacies. They also charged that the process used to develop the program was illegal and that the program was developed with input from PBMs but not from community pharmacy.

The growth of managed care has resulted in numerous changes in channels.

Community pharmacy organizations have also sought legislation to require that PBMs be regulated by state boards of pharmacy or insurance commissioners, to ban economic incentives that encourage use of mail order pharmacy, and to require a standard format and information on prescription drug cards.

SUMMARY

Channels of distribution are the paths through which goods, and information and payment for those goods, travel on their way from manufacturer to ultimate consumer. Traditionally, pharmaceutical channels consisted of manufacturers, wholesalers, and pharmacies. Goods moved from manufacturers to wholesalers to pharmacies to consumers, and payment for goods moved in the opposite direction. The growth of managed care has resulted in numerous changes in channels. The most important of these include the development of PBMs as a channel for payment and information flow, increased cooperation among community pharmacies, consolidation of community pharmacies, and increased conflict between community pharmacies and other channel members.

References

1. *2006 Industry Profile.* Washington, DC: Pharmaceutical Research and Manufacturers of America; 2006.
2. Biotechnology Industry Association. Biotechnology Industry Facts. Available at: www.bio.org/speeches/pubs/er/statistics.asp?p=yes. Accessed May 23, 2007.
3. Generic Pharmaceutical Association. About generics—statistics. Available at: www.gphaonline.org/Content/NavigationMenu/AboutGenerics/Statistics/default.htm. Accessed December 1, 2006.
4. Healthcare Distribution Management Association. The vital link in distribution. Available at: www.healthcaredistribution.org/press_room/pdf/vitallink_092705.pdf. Accessed December 1, 2006.
5. Healthcare Distribution Management Association. 2005–2006 HDMA Factbook: Industry Overview. Arlington, Va: HDMA Foundation; 2006.
6. Miller L. The chain pharmacy industry profile—2006. Alexandria, Va: NACDS Foundation; 2006.
7. Healthcare Distribution Management Association. Healthcare product distribution: a primer. Available at: www.HealthcareDistribution.org. Accessed April 3, 2002.

8. Wentz WH. One lawyer's view of discriminatory pricing. *Am Pharm.* 1994; NS34:24–42.

9. Flanagan ME. Discriminatory pricing lawsuits could change future of community pharmacy. *Am Pharm.* 1994;NS34:20–2.

10. Slezak M. Steering the market toward generics. *Am Drug.* 1997; 214(11): 42–7.

11. Vaczek D. Plans squeeze generic profitability. *Am Drug.* 1995;212(5):40–5.

12. Winslow R, Martinez B. Pharmacy-benefit managers launch aggressive bids to lower drug costs. *Wall Street Journal.* August 20, 2001.

13. Fuhrmans V. Employers, insurers push generics harder. *Wall Street Journal.* October 31, 2006.

14. Ascione FJ, Kirking DM, Gaither CA, et al. Historical overview of generic medication policy. *J Am Pharm Assoc.* 2001;41:567–77.

15. Ukens C. Squaring off: narrow therapeutic index drugs ignite battles. *Drug Top.* 2002;146(7):105.

16. Harris G, Adams C. Drug manufacturers are intensifying courtroom attacks that slow generics. *Wall Street Journal.* July 12, 2001.

17. Conlan MF. Drug firms spent big on lobbying in first half of '96. *Drug Top.* 1996;140(22):60–2.

18. Salzman C. Mandatory monitoring for side effects: the "bundling" of clozapine. *N Engl J Med.* 1990;323:827–30.

19. Glaser M. Off limits: the growth of pharmaceuticals bearing restrictions has the profession and pharmacists worried. *Drug Top.* 2001:145(5):57–65.

20. Gold R. Drug makers win Medicaid fight in possible sign of coming battles. *Wall Street Journal.* August 20, 2001.

21. Hensley S, Cafrey A, Gold R. Drug industry launches effort to block limits on prescriptions. *Wall Street Journal.* March 11, 2002.

22. Zarowitz BJ, Muma B, Coggan P, et al. Managing the pharmaceutical industry-health system interface. *Ann Pharmacother.* 2001;35:1661–8.

23. Health Industry Group Purchasing Association. About HIGPA. Available at: www.higpa.org/about/about_faqs.asp. Accessed December 5, 2006.

24. Federation of Pharmacy Networks. Who we are. Available at: www.fpn. org/who.htm. Accessed December 5, 2006.

25. *Managed Care Digest Series 2005: HMO-PPO/ Medicare-Medicaid Digest.* Bridgewater, NJ: sanofi aventis; 2005.

26. McKesson. Third-party contracting. Available at: www.mckesson. com/en_us/McKesson.com/For%2BPharmacies/Retail%2BNationa l%2BChains/Managed%2BCare/AccessHealth%2BServices/Third-Party%2BContracting.html. Accessed November 15, 2006.

27. Health Mart Pharmacy. Available at: www.healthmart.com/fbenefits.php. Accessed November 15, 2006.

28. AmerisourceBergen. GNP welcomes 2,500th member. Insights Newsletter, 6(9):1, September 2006. Available at: www.amerisourcebergen.com/ cp/1/news_events/insights.jsp. Accessed November 15, 2006.

29. AmerisourceBergen. [Insert Family Pharmacy.] Available at www. amerisourcebergen.com/cp/1/tools/search.jsp?col=abccust&qt=family+pharmacy. Accessed November 15, 2006.

30. AmerisourceBergen. Third Party Network. Available at: www.ameri-sourcebergen.com/cp/1/markets/retail_pharmacies/independent/patient_care/perform_plus/index.jsp. Accessed November 15, 2006.
31. Cardinal Health. Leader pharmacies. Available at: www.cardinal.com/us/en/pharmacies/community/distribution/leader/index.asp. Accessed November 15, 2006.
32. Smith C, Cowan C, Heffler S, et al. National health spending in 2004: recent slowdown led by prescription drug spending. *Health Aff.* January 2006;25:186–96.
33. Stefano S, Navarro RP. The role of the pharmaceutical industry in managed health care. In: Navarro RP, ed. *Managed Care Pharmacy Practice.* Gaithersburg, Md: Aspen; 2002:433–47.
34. *Prescription Drug Benefit Cost and Plan Design Survey Report.* Tempe, Ariz: Pharmacy Benefit Management Institute, Inc: 2005.
35. Pharmaceutical Care Management Association. The value of mail service. Available at: www.pcmanet.org. Accessed April 17, 2002.
36. Express Scripts. Mail service pharmacy. Available at: www.express-scripts.com. Accessed April 17, 2002.
37. *The Merck-Medco Drug Trend Report.* Franklin Lakes, NJ: Merck-Medco Managed Care, LLC; 2001.
38. Carroll NV, Brusilovsky I, York B, et al. Comparison of the costs of community and mail service pharmacy. *J Am Pharm Assoc.* 2005;45:336-43.
39. *The Takeda and Lilly Prescription Drug Benefit Cost and Plan Design Survey Report: 2001 Edition.* Scottsdale, Ariz: Pharmacy Benefit Management Institute, Inc: 2001.
40. Henderson RR, Motheral BR. Mail-order pharmacy: a case study. *Drug Benefit Trends.* 2001:13(9):28–8.
41. *Class-of-Trade Analysis: A Pharmaceutical Market Overview Using IMS/DDD Data.* Totowa, NJ: IMS America; 1992.
42. About NISPC. Available at: www.nispcnet.org/about_NISPC.html. Accessed March 30, 2007.
43. National Community Pharmacists Association. Community pharmacy groups form SureScript Systems to provide electronic connectivity link between prescribers and pharmacists. Available at: www.ncpanet. org. Accessed April 11, 2002.
44. Top 25 drug chains by store count. *Chain Drug Review.* April 23, 1990.
45. Conlan MF. Pharmacy's day in court. *Drug Top.* 1996:140(10):48–58.
46. Meinhardt RA. The Medicare drug discount card program: its structure and the pending lawsuit. *Drug Benefit Trends.* 2001:13(9):15–21.

Additional Readings

Carroll NV. Changes in channels of distribution: wholesalers and pharmacies in organized health-care settings. *Hosp Pharm Rep.* 1997;11:48–57.
Carroll NV. The effects of managed care on the retail distribution of pharmaceuticals. *Manag Care Interface.* 1998;11(11):105–13.

Carroll NV. Examining the rift between the pharmaceutical industry and the pharmacy profession: a channels of distribution approach. *J Pharm Mark Manage.* 2007; in press.

Churchill GA Jr, Peter JP. Managing distribution channels. In: Churchill GA Jr, Peter JP, eds. *Marketing: Creating Value for Customers.* Boston: Irwin McGraw-Hill; 1998:364–90.

Garis RI, Clark BE, Siracuse MV, et al. Examining the value of pharmacy benefit management companies. *Am J Health Syst Pharm.* 2004:61:81–5.

Lipton HL, Kreling DH, Collins T, et al. Pharmacy benefit management companies: dimensions of performance. *Annu Rev Public Health.* 1999;30:361–401.

Perreault WD Jr, McCarthy EJ. Place and development of channel systems. In: *Essentials of Marketing: A Global-Managerial Approach.* Boston: Irwin McGraw-Hill; 1997:242–61.

Taniguchi R. Pharmacy benefit management companies. *Am J Hosp Pharm.* 1995;52:1915–7.

Exercises and Questions

1. What are channels of distribution?
2. Compare and contrast channels of distribution for typical pharmaceuticals, jet airliners, and surgery.
3. Explain how a pharmacy benefit manager (PBM) acts as an intermediary. Compare wholesalers and PBMs in their role as intermediaries.
4. Discuss how expanded pharmacy care services may lead to both cooperation and conflict with other health care providers.
5. List five services that PBMs provide and describe whether these services result in conflict or cooperation in the channels of distribution.

Index

Note: Italic *f* indicates material in figures; italic *t* indicates material in tables.

A

AARP pharmacy service, 224–225
academic detailing, 12, 38, 244
access convenience, 139*t*, 189–190
actual buyers, 29
actual market, 30–31, 31*f*
adherence/nonadherence
    factors in, 111
    market segmentation by, 223*t*, 224
administered vertical marketing
    systems, 298
advertising, 244, 245–248
    cooperative, 253
    and need recognition, 114
affective loyalty, 141
age cohorts, 219, 220*t*. *See also* seniors
aging population, 9
alternative therapy use, market
    segmentation by, 209
American Pharmacists Association,
    mission statement of, 155
AmerisourceBergen, 299
apology, for service failure, 96
attitude
    and health behavior, 125
    of service employees, 73, 74*t*, 91
audits
    convenience, 192–193
    service, 102–103, 143*t*
augmented product, 26–27
"authority seekers," 224
average cost of service. *See* Service
    cost(s)

B

baby boomers, 9, 219, 220*t*
backstage employee actions, 97–100,
    98*f*

bad service. *See* poor service
"Band-Aiders," 231
behavior, 4. *See also* consumer
    behavior; health behavior
    control over, 125
    market segmentation by, 225–230
    models of, 124–127
behavior change, transtheoretical
    model of, 126, 229
behavioral data, categories of, 217*t*
behavioral loyalty, 141
behavioral segmentation, 225–230
    by actual behavior, 226–229, 230
    categories and examples, 217*t*
    by potential behavior, 229, 230
beneficiaries, 302
benefits segmentation, 230–231
    categories and examples, 217*t*
biotechnology companies, 290
Boston Consulting Group, 185
brand(s), 167–171
    definition of, 167
    pharmacist as, 167, 170–171, 174
brand awareness, 167–168
    and brand equity, 169*f*
brand equity, 169–170
    model, 169*f*
brand image, 168–169, 170
    and brand equity, 169*f*
    changing, 170–171
brand meaning. *See* Brand image
brand recall, 168
brand recognition, 167–168
branding, 167–171
    checklist, 174
budgetary constraints, on health care
    purchasers, 10
bundling, 285–286
business climate changes, 164*t*